SIRTFOOD DIET

BOOK

The Complete Guide to Kick-Start Your "Skinny Gene", Get Lean Muscle and Burn Fat. Set Out a Healthy Lifestyle Enjoying the Food You Love.

Adele Middleton

Table of Contents

Introduction

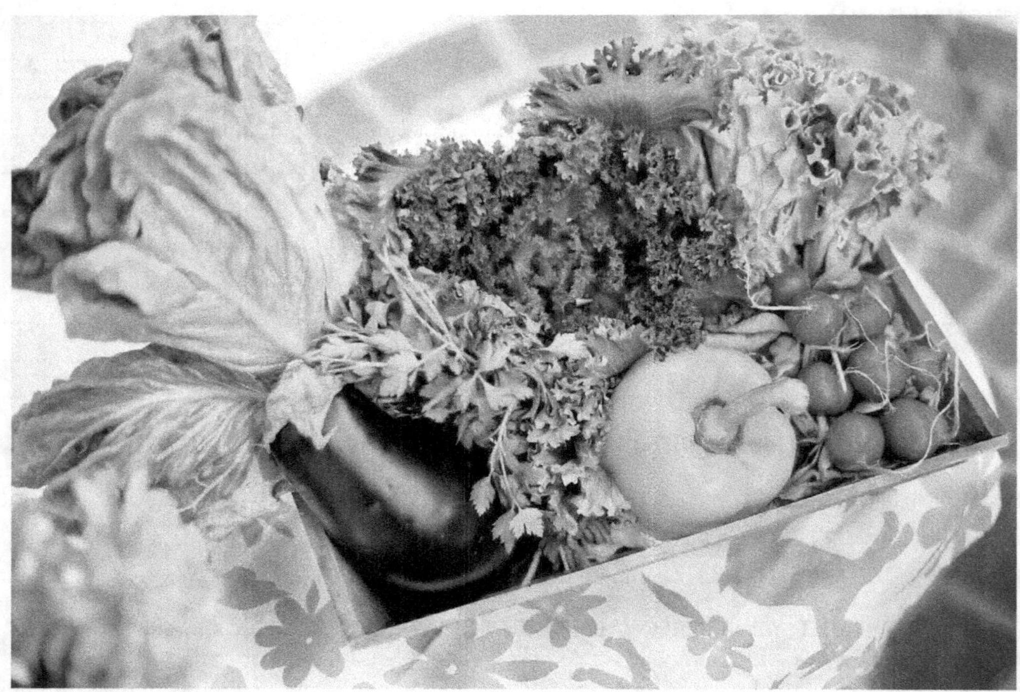

Weight loss is one of the primary concerns of many when it comes to starting to live healthily. This book will guide you in living a healthier life by following the Sirtfood Diet that is based on increasing your metabolism, reducing caloric intake, and improving cell longevity. The Sirtfood Diet was invented by two health consultants, named Dr. Glen Matten and Dr. Aidan Goggins, to help improve weight loss in the short term, but long-term results also include better health overall, such as greatly reducing heart disease, obesity, diabetes, and early death.

Sirtfoods are foods that contain sirtuin-activating compounds which activate a certain family of proteins in your body called sirtuin or SIRT1 protein that works with a group of enzymes in your body to not only make your body burn more fat than usual but also reduce the number of calories that is absorbed into your body. Activated sirtuin also works to aid in improving cell longevity which treats age-related diseases such as hypertension, cancer, osteoarthritis, osteoporosis, type 2 diabetes, and many others. The Sirtfood Diet will help you with successful weight loss that will make you have improved energy and better wellbeing.

The Sirtfood Diet also introduces to us a green juice that will substitute some of your meals within the diet plan. This green juice is made of kale leaves, parsley, celery, green apple, and some other ingredients that are rich in antioxidants and will help cleanse your body to get rid of toxins and free radicals which are molecules produced by our body when it breaks down food.

Why do I need a cookbook for a diet plan?

This cookbook will provide you with easy-to-make recipes that follow the Sirtfood Diet Plan guidelines for your convenience. This will make it so easier for you to follow and stick to the diet plan to give you results that will be satisfactory and will make you happier. This will also improve your cooking skills in addition to being able to live healthily.

How will this diet plan affect me?

The Sirtfood Diet Plan will help you in your weight loss journey and into living a longer and healthier life. It will help you improve your well-being and also teach you to be more disciplined with yourself. These results accompanied by less food restrictions compared to other diet plans will give you the inspiration you need to keep going and stick to the diet plan for a longer period of time.

What should I expect to learn after reading this book?

This book will give you information about Sirtfoods and Sirtuins: what they are, where they come from, what do they do, why you need to incorporate them into your lifestyle, and how to do it.

Chapter 1.   The Science Behind the Sirtfood Diet

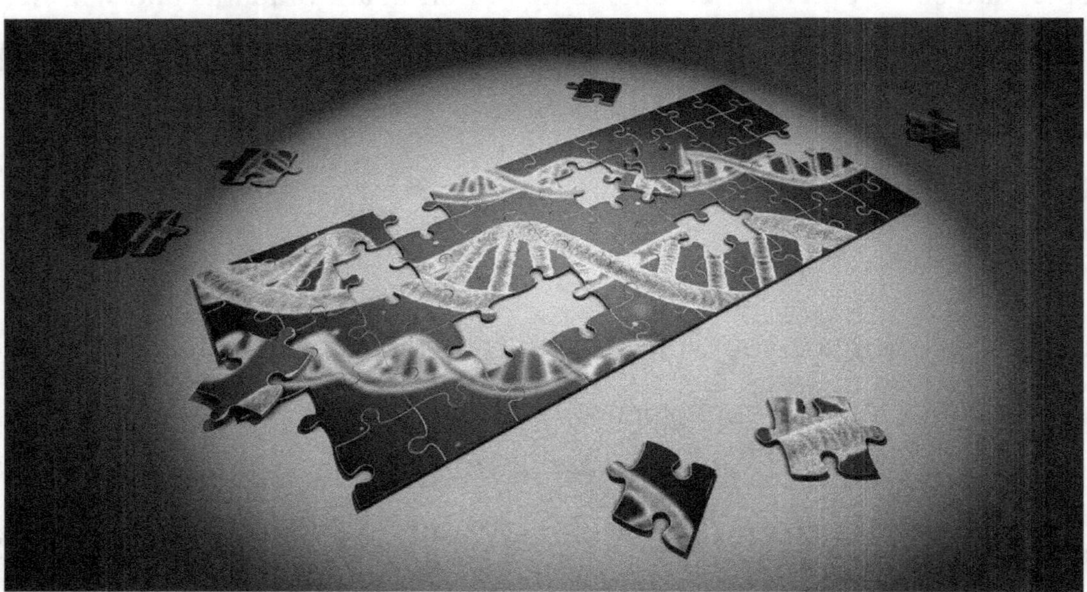

What is the Sirtfood Diet?

The Sirtfood Diet is a ground-breaking diet that gives the ability to turn on an antiquated family of genes that exists in every one of us. The name given to this family of genes is sirtuin. Sirtuins are unique since they orchestrate forms found inside our cells that impact such significant things as our ability to burn fat, our susceptibility to illness, and even our life expectancy. So significant is the impact of sirtuins that they are currently alluded to as "master metabolic regulator." This is precisely what anybody needs to lose a few pounds and carry on with a long and healthy life.

Naturally, sirtuins have become the subject of extreme scientific research lately. The first sirtuin was found in 1984 in yeast, and intrigued interest that truly took off through the span of the following three decades when it was uncovered that sirtuin activation improves life span, first in yeast, and afterward in mice.

From yeast to human beings and every other organism in between, the essential standards of cell metabolism are indistinguishable. In the event that you can control something as modest as growing yeast and see an advantage, at that point rehash it in higher living beings, for example, mice, the potential exists for similar advantages to be acknowledged in people.

Sirtuins, as prior said are, an ancient family of genes with the ability to assist us with burning fat, forming muscle, and keeping us super healthy. It is settled that sirtuins can be turned on through caloric limitation, fasting, and exercise; however, there is another progressive method to accomplish this: food. We consider the foods that generally aid in enacting sirtuins as Sirtfoods.

As such, we can consider every new diet through a prism of positive skepticism. The latest to generate news is the Sirtfood Diet, which will assist with weight loss and other advantages such as "stimulating rejuvenation and cellular recovery" if we are to accept arguments at face value.

This sounds good – and Sirtuin is generally active in a broad range of cellular processes, including aging, growth, and the circadian rhythm. The diet is often partially focused on limiting calories. The nutritionists behind this suggest the diet "influences the ability of the body to burn fat and enhance the metabolic system."

And what do we think about the diet? The answer from a scientific point of view is very little. In response to changes in energy levels, Sirtuin contributes to the regulation of fat and glucose metabolism. They can also play a role in improving the impact of calorie restrictions on aging. This may be via the effects of Sirtuin on aerobic (or mitochondrial) metabolism, decreasing species of reactive oxygen (free radicals), and increasing antioxidant enzymes.

Work also shows that transgenic mice with elevated SIRT6 rates live considerably longer than wild-type mice and that improvements in SIRT6 expression could be related to the aging of certain human skin cells. Also, slow metazoan (yeast) aging has been shown in SIRT2. It sounds amazing, and the diet has some positive feedback, but none of this is convincing empirical proof of the Sirtfood Diet having a comparable impact on actual people. Thinking that laboratory work on rodents, yeast, and human stem cells had some effect on real-world health results – contaminated as they are by a plethora of confusing factors – would be a monumental over-extrapolation.

How It Works

Many diets that have become popular in recent times are based on fasting. The Sirt diet, on the other hand, does not provide for a drastic reduction in calories but promises to achieve the same results. Let's see what it consists of.

The diet regime takes its name from sirt1, a protein that would inhibit fat, going to move the metabolism of the fats themselves. Certain foods in particular would be able to speed up weight loss, allowing us to lose up to three and a half pounds a week.

The Sirt diet involves the introduction of a group of very nutrient-rich foods into a daily and healthy diet. This diet is not based on fasting, which in many cases is responsible for a feeling of hunger, irritability, and loss of muscle mass. Sirt foods would have nutrients that can activate the thinness genes, the same that are activated when you fast. These are sirtuins, which became quite identified because of the research conducted in 2003. It was seen that resveratrol, a substance contained in grapes and red wine, would have the same effects that would be obtained with a calorie restriction. Thanks to this study, it was decided that this topic should be investigated to find other foods with the same properties.

Indeed, sirt genes would accelerate their activity by drawing directly from fat and increasing resistance to disease. But in the beginning, it was thought that one should submit to an iron diet. Then, a whole series of foods were discovered which if ingested allow to obtain the same results, associating them with a healthy and balanced diet.

The creators of the Sirtfood Diet claim that the greatest results in terms of weight loss are obtained in the first phase of this diet. In particular, there is talk of a loss of 3.2 kilos in 7 days. A maximum of 1,000 calories per day should be consumed over the first three days. For this, you can consume three green juices and a solid meal, made with Sirt foods. From the fourth to the seventh day, you can eat 1,500 calories daily. For this purpose, you can consume two green juices and two solid meals, always based on Sirt foods. The authors of the diet claim that even if calories are reduced, participants should not feel hungry, because Sirt foods would have a satiating effect.

After the first week, what is called phase 2 will take over. The second phase is the maintenance phase and has a duration of 14 days. Even if the goal in this phase is not to reduce calories, you will continue to lose weight. During these two weeks, you will have to consume three meals a day rich in Sirt foods and a green maintenance juice. The creators of the diet talk about phases that can be repeated from time to time to lose a few pounds. Some may need to repeat them every three months, others even only once a year.

The Discovery and History of Sirtuin

In the 1970s, geneticist Dr. Amar Klara identified the first Sirtuin, dubbed SIR2, defining it as a gene that regulated yeast cells' capacity to fit. Years after, in the 1990s, researchers identified certain genes homologous — identical in function — to SIR2 in other species such as mice, fruit flies, and then called these SIR2 homologs Sirtuin. Every organism had a different number of Sirtuin. For example, yeast has five Sirtuin, one has bacteria, seven have mice, and seven have humans.

In 1991, alongside graduate students, Nick Austria and Brian Kennedy, Elysium co-founder, and MIT biologist Leonard Guarantee performed experiments to better grasp how yeast agreed. By mistake, Austria decided to cultivate colonies of various yeast strains from samples that he had kept for months in his fridge, causing a hostile atmosphere for the strains. Just a few of these strains will grow here, but a pattern was identified by Guarantee and his team: the longest-lived strains of yeast that survived the best in the fridge. This offered Guarantee instructions so that he could concentrate exclusively on certain long-living yeast strains.

That led to SIR2 being identified as a gene that promoted yeast longevity. There is also no current evidence that this work can be extrapolated to people, and more research on the effects of SIR2 on people is needed. The Guarantee lab thus observed that eliminating SIR2 significantly reduced yeast life, while, most notably, raising the number of copies of the SIR2 gene from one to two expanded the yeast life period. But, naturally, what activated SIR2 had yet to be found.

It is here where the acetyl classes come into action. Initially, it was thought that SIR2 could be a deacetylation enzyme — meaning it removed those acetyl groups — from other molecules, but nobody knew if this was true, because all try to show this operation was negative in the test tube. In Guarantee's own words: "SIR2 does nothing without the NAD+." That was the crucial discovery of Sirtuin biology on the arc.

Benefits of Sirtuin

By actuating our old sirtuin genes we can burn fat and construct a more slender and healthier body. What's more, with sirtuins at the center of our metabolism and, their significance stretches out a long way past body components alone, to each feature of our healthiness.

Think about an ailment that you associate with getting old and the odds are an absence of sirtuin movement in the body is included. For instance, sirtuin initiation is extraordinary for heart health, securing the muscle cells in the heart, and for the most part, helping the heart work better. It likewise improves how our bodies work, causes us to handle cholesterol all the more proficiently and secures against the stopping up of our veins and arteries known as atherosclerosis.

Sirtuin enactment expands the measure of insulin that can be discharged and causes it to work all the more successfully in the body. As it occurs, one of the most famous antidiabetic drugs, metformin, depends on SIRT1 for its valuable impact. To be sure, one pharmaceutical organization is currently exploring adding sirtuin activators to metformin treatment for diabetics, with results demonstrating an amazing 83 percent decrease in the portion of metformin required for similar impacts.

With regards to the brain, sirtuins are included once more, with sirtuin movement seen as lower in Alzheimer's patients. Interestingly, sirtuin activation improves correspondence flags in the cerebrum, upgrades intellectual ability, and lessens mind aggravation. This stops the development of amyloid-β creation and tau protein accumulation, two of the fundamental harming things we see happening in the cerebrums of Alzheimer's patients.

Osteoblasts are exceptional cells in our bones responsible for building new bone. The more osteoblasts we have, the stronger our bones. Sirtuin enactment advances the creation of osteoblast cells, yet also builds their endurance. This makes sirtuin initiation basic for long-lasting bone health.

Malignant growth has been a progressively dubious region for sirtuin studies, and keeping in mind that ongoing examination shows that sirtuin enactment assists with stifling disease tumors, researchers are just barely starting to disentangle this intricate field. While there is considerably more to learn on this specific point, those societies that eat the most Sirtfoods have the least malignancy rates, as we will before long observe.

Heart diseases, diabetes, dementia, osteoporosis, and likely cancer: it's a noteworthy list of infections that can be forestalled by initiating sirtuins. It might not shock discover that societies previously eating a lot of Sirtfoods as a major aspect of their conventional weight control plans experience a life span and healthiness a large portion of us could scarcely envision, which you'll hear more on very soon.

That leaves us with an energizing end: basically, by including the world's most intense Sirtfoods to your diet, and making that a deep-rooted propensity, you also can encounter this degree of healthiness—and that's only the tip of the iceberg—all while getting the build you need.

Benefits of the Sirtfood Diet

While it is still not fully researched and explored, the evidence currently points out that there is a wide range of benefits to the use of sirtuin activation. You can see all sorts of dietary benefits to this particular regimen that will overall make you a much healthier person. Currently, it is believed that you can find all sorts of real, compelling benefits if you make use of this diet on a regular basis, and that is promising. Let's go over some of the most common benefits now, and keep in mind that as of now, there is evidence to suggest this, but more research will need to be done over time.

You Will Lose Weight

The most obvious of the benefits is that you will lose weight on this diet. Whether you are exercising or not, there is no way that you would not lose weight when you follow the diet diligently. This diet will have you restrict your calories enough that anyone would lose weight. The average person uses around 2000 calories per day, and this diet will work to have you cut that in half; you will be providing yourself with just 1000 or 1500 calories based on the phase that you are in.

Weight loss is caused by a calorie deficit—it is as simple as that. When you restrict your calories, but you keep your metabolism up, you will find that you will naturally lose weight. This is normal. However, usually, that weight loss is a mix of fat and muscle. As you lose weight and muscle, you would then naturally see your metabolism slow as well. Of course, this means that over time, your weight loss plan is not nearly as effective as it was supposed to be, and as a direct result, you will have to cut calories further to keep that deficit between consumed calories and the calories that your body naturally burns. This means that weight loss eventually slows, or even plateaus if all you do is make use of a weight-loss regimen through cutting calories. You will lose muscle if you are not careful with the weight loss regimen and that will work against you.

However, thanks to the fact that you do not lose muscle mass during the Sirtfood Diet, you do not have to worry about this problem; you simply continue to lose weight because you are able to maintain your metabolism at levels that will be conducive to you continuing to lose that weight.

Your Appetite Will Slow

Though your first few days you may find that you are ravenous as your body adjusts to its new normal, over time, you should find that your diet will begin to slow down. Your body will adjust to the restrictions in calories, and you will be okay with the lower calorie days, especially because the food that you will be eating will include nutrient-dense food that will help your body feel like it is more satisfied. Lentils and buckwheat are very dense foods that are featured heavily in this diet, and you are able to add healthy fats, such as olive oil, to your diet so that you can feel truly satisfied, knowing that ultimately, you have given yourself enough to keep your body going. You will find that you will be able to tolerate the lower amounts of food, and that is a huge plus.

Does the Sirtfood Diet Actually Work?

There is by all accounts a developing number of famous people and remarkable figures who've touted the Sirtfood Diet for their ongoing weight loss achievement. Be that as it may, buyers must remember that famous people often approach proficient help when it comes to what they devour and any extra exercise regimens. Also, studies on the adequacy of this diet are thin. Without a doubt, most nourishments recorded are solid entire nourishment alternatives and calorie limitations which are consequently associated with some weight loss. Most of the nourishments recorded have mitigating properties, high measures of cancer prevention agents, and supplements which are obviously helpful. Therapeutic specialists caution, however, that while snappy weight loss is conceivable on such a diet, a larger part of that underlying loss will be water weight. It might likewise be hazardous for the individuals who take part in moderate to high physical movement.

While regimens like the Sirtfood Diet still can't seem to be demonstrated when it comes to feasible weight loss, restorative weight loss is a demonstrated and successful answer for any individual who has battled with weight changes and cycles. Diet Demand's primary care physician planned diets are altered to every person for protected, quickened results that lead to long haul achievement.

The most recent diet furor that is slanting among superstars is the Sirtfood Diet. The diet was brought to the spotlight by two VIP nutritionists in the UK who asserted it as a progressive new diet that works by turning on your "thin quality." According to their case, the Sirtfood Diet can advance quick weight loss while keeping up bulk and keep you from constant sickness.

Sirtfoods and Their Nutrients

While all plants have these pressure reaction structures, just certain ones have been created to deliver significant measures of sirtuin-enacting polyphenols. We call these plants Sirtfoods. Their disclosure implies that rather than fasting or laborious exercise programs, there is presently a progressive better approach to initiate your sirtuin genes: eating a diet with adequate Sirtfoods.

It's so flawlessly straightforward, so natural and this is the means by which nature proposed us to eat, instead of the stomach rumbling or calorie tallying of present-day slimming down. Recall this: the cutting-edge way to deal with diet is just 150 years of age; Sirtfoods were created naturally in excess of a billion years prior.

Furthermore, with that, you're presumably tingling to comprehend what explicit foods consider Sirtfoods. So right away, here are the best twenty Sirtfoods and their nutrients:

SIRTFOOD	NUTRIENT
Arugula	Quercetin, kaempferol
Chilies	Luteolin, myricetin
Buckwheat	Rutin
Capers	Kaempferol, quercetin
Celery	Apigenin, luteolin
Cocoa	Epicatechin
Coffee	Caffeic acid
Extra virgin olive oil	Oleuropein, hydroxytyrosol
Garlic	Ajoene, myricetin
Green tea	Epigallocatechin gallate (EGCG)
Kale	Kaempferol, quercetin
Medjool dates	Gallic acid, caffeic acid

Parsley	Apigenin, myricetin
Red endive	Luteolin
Red onion	Quercetin
Red wine	Resveratrol, piceatannol
Soy	Daidzein, formononetin
Strawberries	Fisetin
Turmeric	Curcumin
Walnuts	Gallic acid
Buckwheat	Rutin
Capers	Kaempferol, quercetin
Celery	Apigenin, luteolin
Cocoa	Epicatechin
Coffee	Caffeic acid
Extra virgin olive oil	Oleuropein, hydroxytyrosol
Garlic	Ajoene, myricetin
Green tea	Epigallocatechin gallate (EGCG)
Kale	Kaempferol, quercetin
Medjool dates	Gallic acid, caffeic acid

Parsley	Apigenin, myricetin
Red endive	Luteolin
Red onion	Quercetin
Red wine	Resveratrol, piceatannol
Soy	Daidzein, formononetin
Strawberries	Fisetin
Turmeric	Curcumin
Walnuts	Gallic acid

Pros & Cons of Sirtfood Diet

The greatest pro is that this lifestyle strongly promotes red wine, dark chocolate, and coffee, and that's not something you always read!

The compounds which make up our favorite treats are rich in activators of Sirtuin. Though drinking a kale smoothie, of course, followed by a whole bar of Green and Blacks will not see you dropping the pounds. Everything in balance. Aiden and Glen claim attendees never feel hunger – which suggests it's perfect for someone who can't get through a regular cleanse day without feeling like they're going to die because they do not have a Big Mac right away.

The Plan's first week is pretty intense. Days one and three are the most concentrated with a maximum calorie consumption of 1000 – a mixture of three drinks and one dinner. Days four to seven are marginally lenient with an average calorie of 1,500 calories a day. A few of the pros & cons are as below:

Pros:

- The 'sirt foods' are meant to activate your body's Sirtuin, which is a form of protein that helps prevent your cells from dying and contracting diseases and controls your metabolism.
- It is based on a survey carried out by 40 gym-goers who each shed on average 7 lb. in a week without losing muscle mass.
- You should frequently have small doses of dark chocolate and champagne, without feeling guilty!
- This is built to be long-term and to maintain you alive for life and to delay the aging cycle.

Cons:

- For the first week, this is a calorie limit that would undoubtedly cause some people to lose weight regardless of what food is consumed. This means that the subjects could be gaining weight owing to the calorie limitation itself. You only eat 1,000 calories a day over the first three days, while the four days are 1,500 calories a day.
- Restricting your calorie consumption dramatically can be harmful when your body is accustomed to it and can render you feel lethargic.
- There is not enough proof that its claims, particularly the enhancement of your metabolism, carry through. 40-person research is not big enough to suggest it would necessarily act as a safe way to lose weight.
- Just items including 'sirt juices,' green tea, rocket, soy, and walnuts may be on the sirt food list.
- Less focus is put on bringing a range of foods into your diet so you can look and sound fantastic. Feeding a rainbow of fruit and veg every day, for example, means you bring a range of vitamins and minerals into your diet.

The Sirtfood Diet is full of nutritious foods, but eating habits are not pleasant. This hypothesis and safety arguments are, not to mention, founded on large extrapolations from sparse empirical facts. However, it isn't a terrible thing to attach any sort of products to the diet and might even provide certain health benefits.

Who Can Do the Sirtfood Diet?

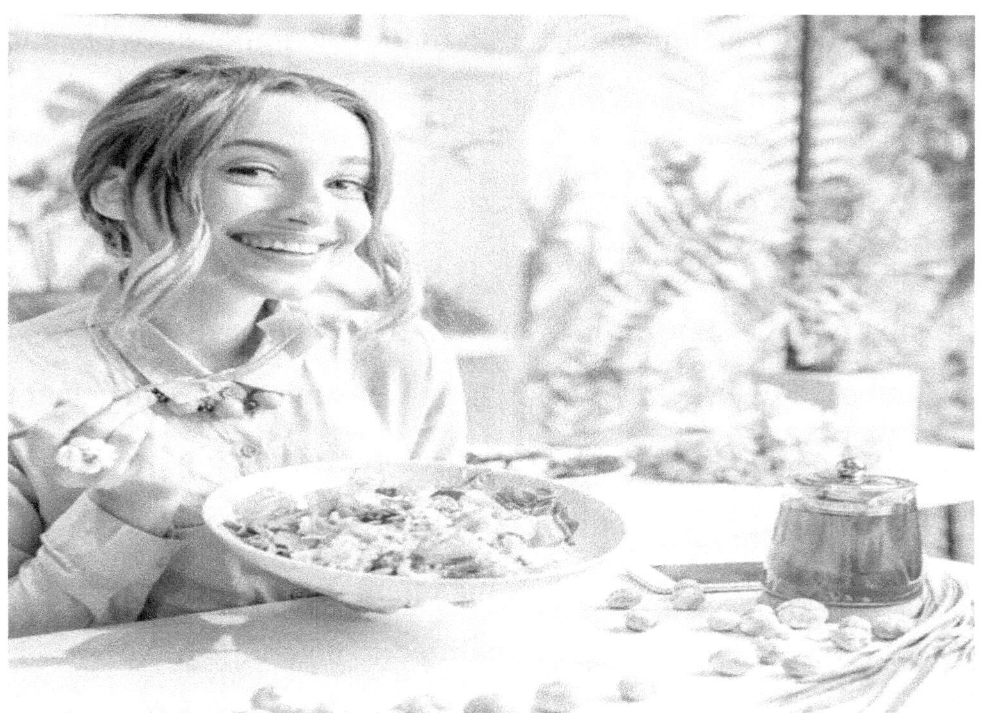

<u>Who Should Try the Sirtfood Diet?</u>

The Sirtfood Diet is suitable for individuals who:

- Are overweight or obese
- Want to maintain his/her weight
- Need to have a "detox" and flush away the toxins from the body
- Have failed to lose weight using different diet techniques
- Want not only to lose weight but also build muscle
- Want a healthier lifestyle and to achieve optimal health

<u>Sirt Diet Safety and Potential Side Effects</u>

Foods rich in sirtuins are also incredibly helpful superfoods that anyone could benefit from eating more of. They are high in anti-inflammatory properties and antioxidants, both of which can reduce the risk of disease and slow down cellular aging. But, if you only choose to eat foods on the Sirt food list that I provided you above, then you will not be eating a balanced diet. This is why the recipes in this book also include other fruits, vegetables, grains, and protein sources. You cannot live off of only a handful of ingredients, at least not healthfully. If you try to eat only sirtuin-rich foods, you may lose more health in the short-term, but you will only experience negative long-term side effects. This is why I, again and again, promote the importance of eating a balanced Sirtfood Diet.

The first phase of the Sirt diet can be restrictive, as you are eating one thousand to fifteen hundred calories a day. However, for this reason, the first phase only lasts a week and is healthy to do in the short-term. You wouldn't want to live an entire month eating that number of calories a day, but, for a week most, it is sufficient for most people. Regularly consult your family doctor before making big life changes that affect your health. Depending on your specific health, weight, and activity level, you might need to make an adjustment to a diet plan to make it work for your individual needs. Your doctor is the one most qualified to determine if you need to make these given adjustments. For instance, if you work a manual labour job, your doctor might recommend you increase your calorie and protein intake to keep your energy levels up. Remember, if your doctor does have concerns due to your individual health, it doesn't mean you can't follow the Sirt diet, simply that you need to make their recommended adjustments to your plan.

Thankfully, the average healthy adult is unlikely to have any problems with the Sirt diet if they follow it in a balanced manner recommended. This means you shouldn't increase the duration of phase one to promote further weight loss. Remember, if you want to lose more weight, then only repeat phase one after completing phase two.

For a healthy adult, the most common side effects are fatigue, irritability, and light-headedness. This is usually due to calorie restriction and can occur whenever a person goes on a diet or changes their eating habits.

You should also know that this diet is not recommended for anyone with an eating disorder. This is because while the calorie restriction is healthy when followed according to plan, for a person who already has disordered eating, it only reinforces their negative relationship with food. The result could be that if someone with an eating disorder attempts to follow this or any other diet calling for counting calories that their eating disorder will likely worsen. Of course, if you or someone you know has an eating disorder and still wants to benefit from Sirtuin-rich foods, you can still enjoy the recipes in this book and incorporate the top Sirtfoods into your daily meal plan without cutting your calorie intake. You may not experience as much weight loss, but you have to prioritize your mental health and healing from disordered eating.

To sum it up, you should speak with your doctor before drastically changing your eating habits no matter what diet you are trying and that includes the Sirt diet. However, if you are healthy and not pregnant, breastfeeding, or suffering from an eating disorder, it should be safe if you follow the diet as recommended. Even if you have a chronic illness or disease, it may be healthy, but only your doctor can say for sure, as each person's disease, condition, and treatment will vary.

Chapter 2.   Dr. Glen Matten and Dr. Aidan Goggins

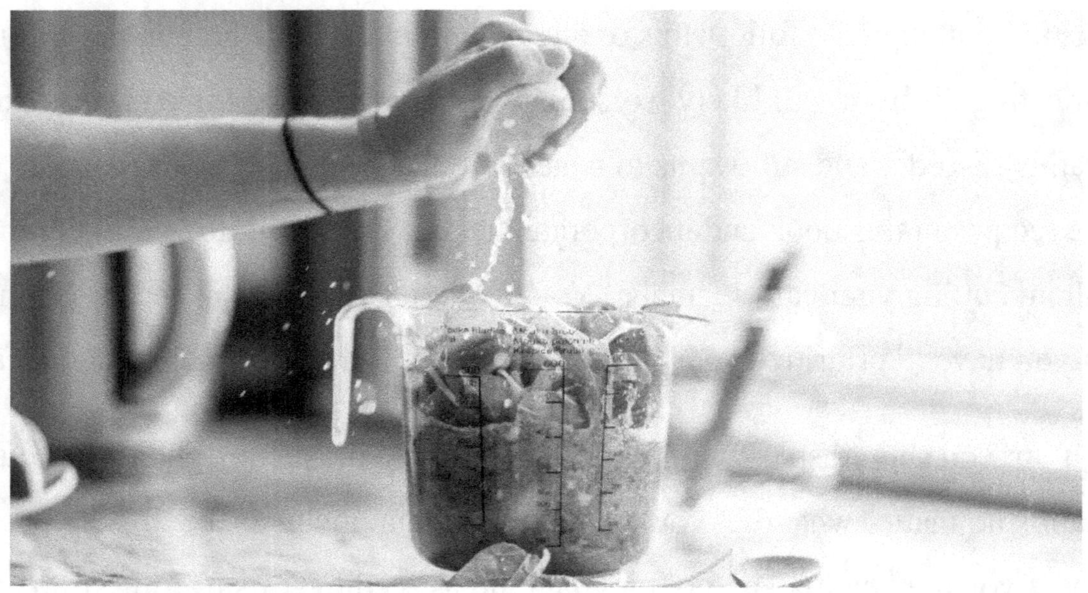

There are two health consultants and authors who invented the Sirtfood Diet. Goggins and Matten hired 37 members from KX Gym in London to check the diet on a broader scale, of whom 15 were overweight. All had performed a small amount of exercise; none had raised it, and some have even continued to do less. The findings were impressive in just one week. Even with the calorie restriction, the test subjects lost an average of 3 kg of fat but put on about 0.8 kg of muscle. With a standard diet that reduces calories in a week by the same amount, you would expect a maximum loss of 1 kg.

They also state that members seldom feel hungry – which implies it's useful for any individual who can't overcome one day of an ordinary wash down without feeling like they are going to black out unless they eat a Big Mac right away. The primary seven day stretch of the arrangement is truly in-your-face. Days one to three are generally escalated with your calorie admission restricted to 1000 – consolidated of three juices and one dinner. Days four to seven are somewhat more indulgent with a calorie limit of 1,500 calories for each day.

Aidan and Glen express that, so as to battle the fasting time frame, you must not concentrate on how much weight you are losing, rather take a gander at the well-being sway on your tone and how your garments fit, and also at how brilliant your skin will look. They also encourage fasters to spread the juices out for the duration of the day instead of having them excessively near one another. Expend the juices, in any event, an hour or two before and after dinners and do not eat any later than 7 p.m.

Nutrition Medicine and Their Brilliant Health Plan

Their health plan is divided into phases:

<u>Phase 1</u>

This phase goes on for seven days. During the initial three days of the diet, you'll drink three Sirtfood squeezes and have one Sirtfood-rich dinner for a day-by-day aggregate of 1,000 calories. On days four through seven, you will devour 1,500 complete calories, drink two green squeezes, and eat two solid Sirtfood-rich suppers. This finishes Phase 1. Phase 1 of the diet is the one that produces the greatest results. Over the course of seven days, you will follow a simple method in order to lose 3.5 kg. Following, you will find a step-by-step guide, complete with menus and recipes.

During the first three days, the intake of calories will have to be limited to one thousand per day at most. Basically, you can have three green juices and a solid meal, all based on Sirt foods. From day 4 to 7, the daily calories will become fifteen hundred. Every day you will eat two green juices and two solid Sirt meals. By the end of the seven days, you should have lost, on average, 3.5 kilos.

Despite the reduction in calories, the participants do not feel hungry, and the calorie limit is an indication rather than a goal. Even in the most intensive phase, calorie restriction is not as drastic as in many other regimes. Sirt foods have a naturally satiating effect so that many of you will feel pleasantly full and satisfied.

Phase 2 is the maintenance phase and lasts 14 days: during this period, although the main objective is not the reduction of calories, you will consolidate weight loss and continue to lose weight. The secret to succeeding at this stage lies in continuing to eat Sirt foods in abundance; following the program that we will provide you with relative recipes will facilitate you. During those two weeks, you will consume three balanced and rich Sirt foods per day and a green Sirt juice.

Phase 2

Phase 2 lasts 14 days and permits you to eat three adjusted Sirtfood-rich dinners and one green juice every day. After Phase 2 is finished, you'll follow a progressively ordinary method for eating, however, are urged to fuse sirtuin-actuating nourishments into normal supper plans. You can return to Phases 1 and 2 whenever you have to lose more weight or muscle to fat ratio.

Monday: 3 green juices

- Breakfast: water + tea or espresso + a cup of green juice
- Lunch: green juice
- Snack: a square of dark chocolate
- Dinner: Sirt meal
- After dinner: a square of dark chocolate

Drink the juices at three distinct times of the day (for example, in the morning as soon as you wake up, mid-morning and mid-afternoon) and choose the normal or vegan dish: pan-fried oriental prawns with buckwheat spaghetti or miso and tofu with sesame glaze and sautéed vegetables (vegan dish).

Tuesday: 3 green juices

- Breakfast: water + tea or espresso + a cup of green juice
- Lunch: 2 green juices before dinner
- Snack: a square of dark chocolate

- Dinner: Sirt meal

- After dinner: a square of dark chocolate

Welcome to day 2 of the Sirtfood Diet. The formula is identical to that of the first day, and the only thing that changes is the solid meal. Today you will also have dark chocolate, and the same goes for tomorrow. This food is so wonderful that we don't need an excuse to eat it.

To earn the title of a "Sirt food", chocolate must be at least 85 percent cocoa. And even among the various types of chocolate with this percentage, not all of them are the same. Often this product is treated with an alkalizing agent (this is the so-called "Dutch process") to reduce its acidity and give it a darker color. Unfortunately, this process greatly reduces the flavonoids activating sirtuins, compromising their health benefits. Lindt Excellence 85% chocolate is not subjected to the Dutch process and is therefore often recommended.

On day 2, capers are also included in the menu. Despite what many may think, they are not fruits, but buds that grow in Mediterranean countries and are picked by hand. They are fantastic Sirt foods because they are very rich in the nutrients kaempferol and quercetin. From the point of view of flavor, they are tiny concentrates of taste. If you've never used them, don't feel intimidated. You will see, they will taste amazingly if combined with the right ingredients, and they will give an unmistakable and inimitable aroma to your dishes.

On the second day, you will intake: 3 green Sirt juices and one solid meal (normal or vegan).

Drink the juices at three distinct times of the day (for example, when you wake up in the morning, mid-morning, and mid-afternoon) and choose either the normal or the vegan dish: Turkey escalope with capers, parsley, and sage on spiced cauliflower couscous or curly kale and red onion dahl with buckwheat (vegan dish)

Wednesday: 3 green juices

- Breakfast: water + tea or espresso + a cup of green juice
- Lunch: 2 green juices before dinner
- Snack: a square of dark chocolate
- Dinner: Sirt meal • After dinner: a square of dark chocolate

You are now on the third day, and even if the format is once again identical to that of days 1 and 2, so the time has come to flavor everything with a fundamental ingredient. For thousands of years, chili has been a fundamental element of the gastronomic experiences of the whole world.

As for the effects on health, we have already seen that its spiciness is perfect for activating sirtuins and stimulating the metabolism. The applications of chili are endless, and therefore represent an easy way to consume Sirt food regularly.

If you are not a big expert on chili, we recommend the bird's eye chili (sometimes called the Thai chili), because it is the best for sirtuins.

This is the last day you will consume three green juices a day; tomorrow, you will switch to two. We, therefore, take this opportunity to browse other drinks that you can have during the diet. We all know that green tea is good for health, and water is naturally very good, but what about coffee? More than half of people drink at least one coffee a day, but always with a trace of guilt because some say that it is a vice and an unhealthy habit. This is absolutely untrue; studies show that coffee is a real treasure trove of beneficial plant substances. That's why coffee drinkers run the least risk of getting diabetes, certain forms of cancer, and neurodegenerative diseases. Furthermore, not only is coffee, not a toxin, it protects the liver and makes it even healthier!

On the third day, you will intake 3 green Sirt juices and 1 one solid meal (normal or vegan, see below).

Drink the juices at three distinct times of the day (for example, in the morning as soon as you wake up, mid-morning and mid-afternoon) and choose the normal or vegan dish: aromatic chicken breast with kale, red onion, tomato sauce, and chili or baked tofu with harissa on spiced cauliflower couscous (vegan dish).

Thursday: 3 green juices

- Breakfast: water + tea or espresso + a cup of green juice
- Lunch: Sirt food
- Snack: 1 green juice before dinner
- Dinner: Sirt food

The fourth day of the Sirtfood Diet has arrived, and you are halfway through your journey to a leaner and healthier body. The big change from the previous three days is that you will only drink two juices instead of three and that you will have two solid meals instead of one. This means that on the fourth day and the upcoming ones, you will have two green juices and two solid meals, all delicious and rich in Sirt foods. The inclusion of Medjoul dates in a list of foods that promote weight loss and good health may seem surprising. Especially when you think they contain 66 percent sugar.

Sugar has no stimulating properties towards sirtuins. On the contrary, it has well-known links with obesity, heart disease, and diabetes; in short, just at the antipodes of the objectives, we aim to. But industrially refined and processed sugar is very different from the sugar present in a food that also contains sirtuin-activating polyphenols: the Medjoul dates. Unlike normal sugar, these dates, consumed in moderation, do not increase the level of glucose in the blood.

Today we will also integrate chicory into meals. Like with onion, red chicory is better in this case too, but endive, its close relative, is also a Sirt food. If you are looking for ideas on the use of these salads, combine them with other varieties and season them with olive oil: they will give a pungent flavor to milder leaves.

On the fourth day, you will intake: 2 green Sirt juices, 2 solid meals (normal or vegan) Drink the juices at different times of the day (for example the first in the morning as soon as you wake up or in the middle of the morning, the second in the middle of the afternoon) and choose the normal or vegan dishes: muesli Sirt, pan-fried salmon fillet with caramelized chicory, rocket salad, and celery leaves or muesli Sirt and Tuscan stewed beans (vegan dish)

Friday: 2 green juices

- Breakfast: water + tea or espresso + a cup of green juice
- Lunch: Sirt food
- Snack: a green juice before dinner
- Dinner: Sirt food

You have reached the fifth day, and the time has come to add fruits. Due to its high sugar content, fruits have been the subject of bad publicity. This does not apply to berries. Strawberries have a very low sugar content: one teaspoon per 100 grams. They also have an excellent effect on how the body processes simple sugars.

Scientists have found that if we add strawberries to simple sugars, this causes a reduction in insulin demand, and therefore transforms food into a machine that releases energy for a long time. Strawberries are, therefore, a perfect element in diets that will help you lose weight and get back in shape. They are also delicious and extremely versatile, as you will discover in the Sirt version of the fresh and light Middle Eastern tabbouleh.

Miso, made from fermented soy, is a traditional Japanese dish. Miso contains a strong umami taste, a real explosion for the taste buds. In our modern society, we know better monosodium glutamate, artificially created to reproduce the same flavor. Needless to say, it is far preferable to derive that magical umami flavor from traditional and natural food, full of beneficial substances. It is found in the form of a paste in all good supermarkets and healthy food stores and should be present in every kitchen to give a touch of taste to many different dishes.

Since umami flavors enhance each other, miso is perfectly associated with other tasty/umami foods, especially when it comes to cooked proteins, as you will discover today in the very tasty, fast, and easy dishes you will eat.

On the fifth day, you will intake 2 green Sirt juices and 2 solid meals (normal or vegan).

Drink the juices at different times of the day (for example the first in the morning as soon as you wake up or in the middle of the morning, the second in the middle of the afternoon) and choose the normal or vegan dishes: buckwheat Tabbouleh with strawberries, baked cod marinated in miso with sautéed vegetables and sesame or buckwheat and strawberry Tabbouleh (vegan dish), soba (buckwheat noodles) in a miso broth with tofu, celery, and kale (vegan dish).

Saturday: 2 green juices

- Breakfast: water + tea or espresso + a cup of green juice
- Lunch: Sirt food
- Snack: a green juice before dinner
- Dinner: Sirt food

There are no Sirt foods better than olive oil and red wine. Virgin olive oil is obtained from the fruit only by mechanical means, in conditions that do not deteriorate it, so that you can be sure of its quality and polyphenol content. "Extra virgin" oil is that of the first pressing ("virgin" is the result of the second) and therefore has more flavor and better quality: this is what we strongly recommend you use when cooking.

No Sirt menu would be complete without red wine, one of the cornerstones of the diet. It contains the activators of resveratrol and piceatannol sirtuins, which probably explain the longevity and slenderness associated with the traditional French way of life, and which are at the origin of the enthusiasm unleashed by Sirt foods.

Of course, wine contains alcohol, so it should be consumed in moderation. Fortunately, resveratrol can withstand heat well, and therefore can be used in the kitchen. Pinot Noir is many people's favorite grape variety because it contains much more resveratrol than most of the others.

On the sixth day, you will consume 2 green Sirt juices and 2 solid meals (normal or vegan).

Drink the juices at different times of the day (for example, the first in the morning as soon as you wake up or in the middle of the morning, the second in the middle of the afternoon) and choose the normal or vegan dishes: Super Sirt salad and grilled beef fillet with red wine sauce, onion rings, garlic curly kale and roasted potatoes with aromatic herbs or super lentil Sirt salad (vegan dish) and mole sauce of red beans with roasted potato (vegan dish).

Sunday: 2 green juices

- Breakfast: a bowl of Sirt Muesli + a cup of green juice
- Lunch: Sirt food • Snack: a cup of green juice
- Dinner: Sirt food

The seventh day is the last of phase 1 of the diet. Instead of considering it as an end, see it as a beginning, because you are about to embark on a new life, in which Sirt foods will play a central role in your nutrition. Today's menu is a perfect example of how easy it is to integrate them in abundance into your daily diet. Just take your favorite dishes and, with a pinch of creativity, you will turn them into a Sirt banquet.

Walnuts are excellent Sirt food because they contradict current opinions. They have high-fat content and many calories, yet it has been shown that they contribute to reducing weight and metabolic diseases, all thanks to the activation of sirtuins. They are also a versatile ingredient, excellent in baked dishes, in salads, and as a snack, alone.

Pesto is becoming an irreplaceable ingredient in the kitchen because it is tasty and allows you to give personality to even the simplest dishes. The traditional one is made with basil and pine nuts, but you can try an alternative one with parsley and walnuts. The result is delicious and rich in Sirt foods.

We can apply the same reasoning to an easy-to-prepare dish, such as an omelet. The dish has to be the typical recipe appreciated by the whole family, and simple to transform into a Sirt dish with a few little tricks. In our recipe, we use bacon. Why? Simply because it fits perfectly. The Sirtfood Diet tells us what to include, not what to exclude, and this allows us to change our long-term eating habits. After all, isn't that the secret to not getting back the lost pounds and staying healthy?

On the seventh day, you will consume 2 green Sirt juices; 2 solid meals (normal or vegan).

Drink the juices at different times of the day (for example the first in the morning as soon as you wake up or in the middle of the morning, the second in the middle of the afternoon) and choose the normal or vegan dishes: Sirt omelet Sirt and baked chicken breast with walnut and parsley pesto and red onion salad or Waldorf salad (vegan dish) and baked aubergine wedges with walnut and parsley pesto and tomato salad (vegan dish).

During the second phase, there are no calorie restrictions but indications on which Sirt foods must be eaten to consolidate weight loss and not run the risk of getting the lost kilograms back.

After the Two Phases of the Diet

Let's assume that you've managed to finish both phases of the Sirtfood Diet. In this case, allow me to congratulate you on your efforts and dedication to finish it. How are you feeling after the diet? Do you feel more energized? Have you lost a significant amount of weight? Do you feel better about yourself? If the answer to all these questions is yes, then why not stick to this diet?

The Sirtfood Diet is a meal plan you can easily stick to, plus it is very satisfying, especially if it meets your expectations. At the moment, there aren't too many known sirtfood recipes, and this means that you simply can't stick to them for the rest of your life. You need to explore different types and try new food, but you should never try unhealthy foods. I don't care how much you miss fast food; this type of food should never be tried by anyone, not even out of curiosity.

The trick is to eat healthy for the rest of your life. You can try all sorts of meals, different cuisines, but as long as you remain faithful to this principle of eating healthy, you shouldn't gain too much weight or suffer from medical conditions or diseases caused by nutrition. Embrace variety, but don't exaggerate with any meals, regardless of the occasion. Another significant problem is eating irregularly. It is not OK to serve breakfast at noon, lunch at 4:00 p.m., and dinner after 9:00 p.m. It is always great to have these meals within a set timeframe. For instance, having breakfast between 7:00 a.m. and 9:00 a.m. sounds like the right thing to do. Lunch should be served between noon and 2:00 p.m., and dinner between 6:00 p.m. and 8:00 p.m. Discipline is the key to staying healthy, not only when it comes to what you eat but also when you eat.

But let's focus more on what you eat! As a Sirtfood Diet fan, you should be a great fan of other diets as well, especially those that involve fruits and veggies. So, you can go 100 percent vegan, or you can even try Mediterranean meals or an LCHF diet. All these meals have plenty of health benefits and can even help you lose weight. Let's take for instance strawberries, the best source of fisetin. If you want to experience a healthy metabolism and slower aging process, you can consume any sort of berries, not just strawberries. So yes, eat blackberries, blueberries, raspberries, or black currants, as they also have a decent level of sirtuin-activating nutrients.

This is applicable to walnuts as well. Perhaps you want to diversify and try different nuts, not just "the champion nut." So why not eat pecans, chestnuts, pistachios, or even peanuts? They all have more or less sirtuin-activating nutrients, so it would be a shame to ignore them as a potential snack.

Over the last few years, there has been a lot of fuss created over the consumption of grains in different forms, whether we are talking about bread, pastry, pasta, and other processed products. Processing grains is what's causing the issue, as this destroys any sirtuin-activating nutrients in whole grains. Consuming whole grains has health benefits like reduced risk of diabetes, inflammation, heart disease, and cancer. Buckwheat is a pseudo-grain, but this doesn't mean that you need to consume only this food from the grain family. No harm can come to you if you consume whole grains, and apparently, quinoa is a perfectly viable option for a sirtfood. If you need more alternatives for a sirtfood snack, then popcorn is the perfect choice for you.

But don't think that foods like chia seeds or goji berries don't have sirtfood properties. They are perfectly reasonable choices if you want to reap the benefits of sirtfood. If you are looking for more alternatives when it comes to sirtfoods, please check the list below:

Vegetables:

- Artichokes

- Asparagus

- Bok choy/pak choi

- Broccoli

- Frisée

- Green beans

- Shallots

- Watercress

- White onions

- Yellow endive

Fruits:

- Apples

- Blackberries

- Black currants

- Black plums

- Cranberries

- Goji berries

- Kumquats

- Raspberries

- Red grapes

Nuts and seeds:

- Chestnuts

- Chia seeds

- Peanuts

- Pecan nuts

- Pistachio nuts

- Sunflower seeds

Grains and pseudo-grains:

- Popcorn

- Quinoa

- Whole-wheat flour

Beans:

- Fava beans

- White beans (e.g., navy or cannellini)

Herbs and spices:

- Chives

- Cinnamon

- Dill (fresh and dried)

- Dried oregano

- Dried sage

- Ginger

- Peppermint (fresh and dried)

- Thyme (fresh and dried)

Beverages:

- Black tea

- White tea

Most nutritionists don't recommend the consumption of too many carbs since they are so harmful to your body, but you can't go wrong with proteins. Having a high-protein diet is what bodybuilders aim for. Nobody wants to lose muscle mass, unless we are talking about some individual cases, like actors trying to lose weight dramatically for a specific role or some athletes trying to fit in a particular weight category.

In normal cases, most people would like to preserve their muscle mass or to increase it. Combining high-protein ingredients with sirtfood ingredients can have plenty of positive effects on your body. Proteins are made of amino acids and leucine, and this last nutrient can work with sirtuins very well. Leucine has a primary role in changing the cell environment to enhance the activity of sirtuin-activating nutrients. Combining a sirtfood meal with leucine-rich protein seems to be the perfect match. Leucine can be found in seafood, eggs, dairy (cheese, milk), poultry, fish, seafood, and red meat (beef, pork).

Now we all want to increase the protein intake to grow our muscle mass, but it is essential to know how we achieve this goal. Eating meat can help you achieve this goal, but you still have to be careful with it, as massive consumption of this food can increase the risk of cancer. Poultry and fish are less harmful, but if you consume too much red meat, you can increase the risk of having cancer. Even if you exaggerate with dairy products and eggs, this increased consumption can have negative impacts on your health.

However, your diet should not consist only of proteins, as there are plenty of health benefits in the consumption of healthy fats. In fact, the LCHF diets focus on fat intake, as the body burns what you eat: fats. When it comes to healthy fats, the omega-3 ones are among the healthiest. These fats can be found in fish, so make sure you consume salmon, trout, sardines, herring, or mackerel. If you have the chance of eating fresh tuna, it would be great, as you will have the chance to boost your omega-3 intake. The canned version has a significantly lower concentration of omega-3 fats.

Sirtuin Proteins and How They Act

SIRT1, just like other SIRTUINS families, are protein NAD+ dependent deacetylases that are associated with cellular metabolism. All sirtuins, including SIRT1, are important for sensing energy status and in protection against metabolic stress. They coordinate cellular response towards Caloric Restriction (CR) in an organism. SIRT1 is found in diverse locations and allows cells to easily sense changes in the level of energy anywhere in the mitochondria, nucleus, and cytoplasm. They are also associated with metabolic health through the deacetylation of several target proteins such as muscles, liver, endothelium, heart, and adipose tissue.

SIRT1, SIRT6, and SIRT7 are localized in the nucleus where they take part in the deacetylation of customers to influence gene expression epigenetically. SIRT2 is located in the cytosol, while SIRT3, SIRT4, and SIRT5 are located in the mitochondria where they regulate metabolic enzyme activities as well as moderate oxidative stress.

SIRT1, as most studies with regards to metabolism, aid in mediating the physiological adaptation to diets. Several studies have shown the impact of sirtuins on Caloric Restriction. Sirtuins deacetylase non-histone proteins that define pathways involved during the metabolic adaptation when there are metabolic restrictions. Caloric Restriction, on the other hand, causes the induction of expression of SIRT1 in humans. Mutations that lead to loss of function in some sirtuins genes can lead to a reduction in the outputs of caloric restrictions. Therefore, sirtuins have the following metabolic functions:

Regulation of the Liver

The liver regulates the body's glucose homeostasis. During fasting or caloric restriction, glucose level becomes low, resulting in a sudden shift in hepatic metabolism to glycogen breakdown and then to gluconeogenesis to maintain glucose supply as well as ketone body production to mediate the deficit in energy. Also, during caloric restriction or fasting, there is muscle activation and liver oxidation of fatty acids produced during lipolysis in white adipose tissue. For this switch to occur, there are several transcription factors involved to adapt to energy deprivation. SIRT1 intervenes during the metabolic switch to see the energy deficit.

At the initial stage of the fasting that is the post glycogen breakdown phase, there is the production of glucagon by the pancreatic alpha cells to active gluconeogenesis in the Liver through the cyclic amp response element-binding protein (CREB), and CREB regulated transcription coactivator 2 (CRTC2), the coactivator. If the fasting gets prolonged, the effect is canceled out, and is being replaced by SIRT1 mediated CRTC2 deacetylase resulting in targeting of the coactivator for ubiquitin/ proteasome-mediated destruction? SIRT1, on the other hand, initiates the next stage of gluconeogenesis through acetylation and activation of peroxisome proliferator-activated receptor coactivator one alpha, which is the coactivator necessary for fork head box O1. In addition to the ability of SIRT1 to support gluconeogenesis, coactivator one alpha is required during the mitochondrial biogenesis necessary for the liver to accommodate the reduction in energy status. SIRT1 also activates fatty acid oxidation through deacetylation and activation of the nuclear receptor to increase energy production. SIRT1, when involved in acetylation and repression of glycolytic enzymes such as phosphoglycerate mutase 1, can lead to shutting down of the production of energy through glycolysis. SIRT6, on the other hand, can be served as a co-repressor for hypoxia-inducible Factor 1 Alpha to repress glycolysis. Since SIRT6 can transcriptionally be induced by SIRT1, sirtuins can coordinate the duration of time for each fasting phase.

Aside from glucose homeostasis, the liver also overtakes in lipid and cholesterol homeostasis during fasting. When there are caloric restrictions, the synthesis of fat and cholesterol in the liver is turned off, while lipolysis in the white adipose tissue commences. The SIRT1, upon fasting, causes acetylation of steroid regulatory element-binding protein (SREBP) and targets the protein to destroy the ubiquitin-professor system. The result is that fat cholesterol synthesis will repress. During the regulation of cholesterol homeostasis, SIRT1 regulates the oxysterol receptor, thereby assisting the reversal of cholesterol transport from peripheral tissue through upregulation of the oxysterol receptor target gene ATP-binding cassette transporter A1 (ABCA1).

Further modulation of the cholesterol regulatory loop can be achieved via bile acid receptor, that is necessary for the biosynthesis of cholesterol catabolic and bile acid pathways. SIRT6 also participates in the regulation of cholesterol levels by repressing the expression and post-translational cleavage of SREBP1/2, into the active form. Furthermore, in the circadian regulation of metabolism, SIRT1 participates through the regulation of the cell circadian clock.

Mitochondrial SIRT3 is crucial in the oxidation of fatty acid in mitochondria. Fasting or caloric restrictions can result in up-regulation of activities and levels of SIRT3 to aid fatty acid oxidation through deacetylation of long-chain specific acyl-CoA dehydrogenase. SIRT3 can also cause activation of ketogenesis and the urea cycle in the liver.

SIRT1 also adds to the metabolic regulation in the muscle and white adipose tissue. Fasting causes an increase in the level of SIRT1, leading to deacetylation of coactivator one alpha, which in turn causes genes responsible for fat oxidation to get activated. The reduction in energy level also activates AMPK, which will activate the expression of coactivator one alpha. The combined effects of the two processes will give rise to increased mitochondrial biogenesis together with fatty acid oxidation in the muscle.

Chapter 3.   Burn Fat and Preserve Muscle

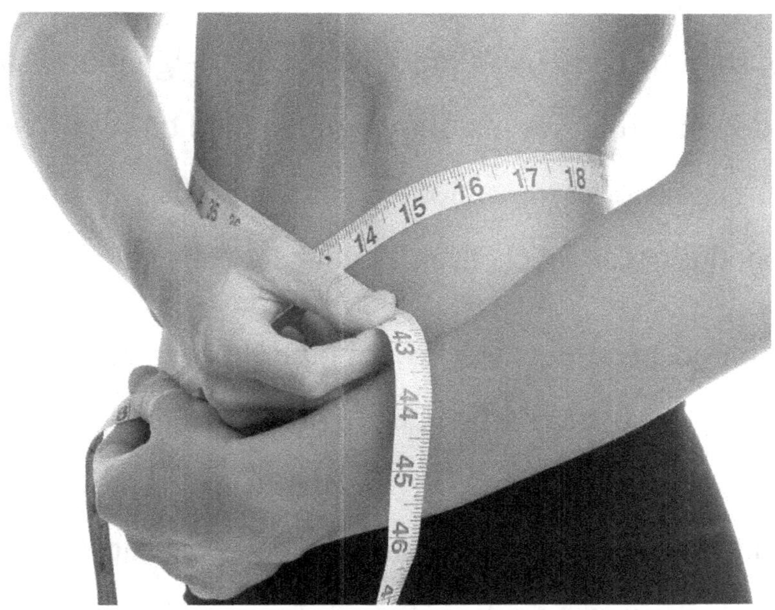

Burn Fat

In addition to protecting your muscles, sirtfoods encourage your metabolic system to start burning through the fat that is stored in your body, which is one of the reasons for the surprising weight loss potential.

Gaining weight is a complex process for humans that involves multiple hormones sending signals back and forth to your various biological processes. One of these hormones is insulin, which I am sure you're familiar with. When you consume any calories, your body needs to convert the food into glucose so that it can be used as energy to keep your body functioning. Some foods, such as sugar or refined carbohydrates, for example, convert to sugar in your bloodstream almost instantaneously, causing a spike in blood glucose levels. Other foods, like complex carbohydrates and proteins, take longer for your body to break down and convert to glucose, so your blood gets a more slow and steady drip of glucose.

When your blood sugar gets too high because you have consumed more sugar than your body needs to operate immediately, it can cause a variety of problems. Headaches, thirst, or fatigue might be experienced in the short-term, but high blood sugar levels can lead to kidney failure, heart disease, or nerve damage if the issue becomes chronic. Obviously, these symptoms are severe and potentially life-threatening, so your body has a process to detect high blood sugar levels and bring them back down: it releases insulin. With the help of your liver and cholesterol, insulin pulls sugar out of your bloodstream and tells your cells to take it in instead and your blood glucose levels drop as your fat cells get a little fuller.

When your blood sugar gets too low, another hormone, glucagon, will be released. Glucagon taps your liver and fat cells in order to release the stored glucose back into your bloodstream. The main problem with our modern diet is that humans have developed the habit of constant grazing and/or over-eating. This provides a constant flow of glucose, triggering a constant need for insulin. Our blood sugar rarely dips low enough to trigger the production of glucagon, so instead of using our stored energy, we simply add more to the reserves.

Swapping a Standard American Diet (SAD) that causes an instant spike in your blood glucose for a Sirtfood Diet will create a slower and steadier flow of energy that will help to reinstate the natural balance of your hormones once again. As an added bonus, studies have shown that activating sirtuins can actually suppress your body's ability to store fat as it increases the propensity to burn it (Picard, et al., 2004). Your metabolic system will actually have a chance to use the stored energy.

Aside from sirtfoods being a more balancing form of energy, by activating our sirtuin genes, our cells are being protected and fortified. Each cell has a power center called a mitochondrion which is responsible for the conversion of glucose into usable energy. This is a lot of work for our cells and, especially if we are eating more calories than we need and those calories are primarily simple carbohydrates, our mitochondria wear out quickly. Sirtuins protect our mitochondria, allowing them to process energy more efficiently. In other words, we can burn fat more quickly.

Sirtfoods work on multiple fronts to help our body naturally regulate weight: they reduce the amount of glucose that gets stored as fat, and they increase the speed at which our fat gets used. As an added bonus, by naturally regulating our metabolism, we can protect ourselves against insulin resistance and type 2 diabetes.

Insulin and glycogen are not the only hormones to return to a healthy balance on a Sirtfood Diet. Leptin is also regulated. Leptin resistance is not as commonly understood as insulin resistance, but it plays just as important of a role in the process of weight gain. Leptin is often called the hunger hormone because it's responsible for telling your brain when you have enough fat stored in your body to keep you safe, and when you need to take in more energy.

If you have low body fat, your brain will throw out hunger signals to encourage you to eat more food. Unfortunately, if you have damaged leptin receptors, your brain will also continue to pump out hunger signals, whether you are actually in need of energy or not. Hunger is hard to ignore, and if your leptin levels are dysregulated, not only are you going to constantly feel hungry, but your body will also be actively trying to store any energy you consume as fat instead of using it immediately.

When you follow a Sirtfood Diet, your leptin levels will naturally balance and your hunger signals will only start to spark when you truly need more nutrition, not simply when your sugar crash has taken a turn for the worse. When all the hormones associated with your metabolism are operating and communicating effectively, you will only store as much body fat as necessary for your health. If you are currently overweight, repairing your metabolic system will help you release weight quickly, until you have reached your optimal body composition.

Preserve Muscle

Sirtuins are genes that activate proteins in your body. Protein is a very popular word in the world of fitness, and we all know that it is absolutely necessary for building the strong muscles that you see gracing the covers of fitness magazines. However, protein is far more important than simply developing bulky muscle mass. Protein is the building block of every single cell in your body.

We all need protein to survive, let alone thrive, and look youthful and strong. Yes, a body that has only lean fat and nicely toned muscles will create an aesthetically pleasing, athletic picture. But muscle is also responsible for holding our skeletons in place, preventing bone loss and joint damage, and keeping our vital organs protected and safe. In fact, our most vital organ, our heart, is a muscle. Just as our muscle protects everything inside our skin, proteins also protect everything inside our cells. Sirtuins insulate our cells and protect them from the damage that a stressful, toxic environment causes. Our bodies are designed to keep us safe, with many different systems of defense in order, but we need to support these systems with the nutrition we consume.

Unfortunately, many of us are starting from a position of current ill-health and probably have a certain amount of excess weight that is causing us difficulty. Muscle and protein are some of the most important factors of shedding that extra body fat.

 Muscle has a much harder job than fat does. Muscle is what allows us to move constantly throughout the day, even if it is just our heart beating. Fat, on the other hand, is designed to simply remain in our bodies, inactive and lazy, until it is needed as an emergency supply of energy. It's not difficult to understand, then, that muscle is going to require a lot more energy to maintain itself. The more muscle you have in your body, the more energy you will burn in a day. This will not only build a strong, healthy body, but it will also accelerate weight loss and promote healthy weight management in the long-term.

Diets that focus exclusively on calorie restriction will force your body to use any energy it finds, and, for a period of time, you will lose weight. That weight will come from a variety of sources, including fat, muscle, and water. If you reach your goal weight, or if you simply return to your normal calorie consumption, your body will refill all the reserves you just emptied, putting all the weight right back on your body.

With the Sirtfood Diet, calorie restriction is limited to a single week, simply to give your body a chance to empty out some of the overwhelm your metabolic system is coping with. After that first week, you will instead be prioritizing the addition of foods that help to activate protein and build healthy muscle cells. This will provide the perfect foundation for complete cellular health, and it will maximize your weight loss efforts until your body naturally returns to its ideal composition.

In the original pilot study during the development stages of the Sirtfood Diet, participants had every morsel of food prepared for them to ensure compliance, and their body composition was monitored every step of the way. It quickly became obvious that, even though the average weight loss was slightly more than 5 pounds in the first week of the diet, muscle mass was not only maintained, but it increased by 1 – 2 pounds.

For those of you who are cringing at the idea of adding any amount of weight to your body, you should realize that muscle, in addition to burning more energy, also takes up less space than fat. This means that if you were to lose 2 pounds of fat and gain 2 pounds of muscle, though the number on the scale will be the same, your body will be physically smaller which, after all, is the primary goal. In regard to the pilot study, if the weight loss were adjusted to reflect muscle gain, the average would be increased to approximately 7 pounds within a single week (Goggins & Matten, 2018).

The scientific reasoning for this extraordinary result is the activation of your sirtuin genes, which guard your cells against protein loss and muscle breakdown. As long as we're activating our sirtuins, even in a caloric deficit, our muscles will be protected and working in our favor. Without the activation of sirtuins, our muscles will actually shrink because they don't have the ability to develop or regenerate when damaged.

It isn't just the size or quantity of muscle that you have in your body that is important, but it is also the biological age of those muscles. One of the cruel realities of growing older is that damage in our body accumulates over the years, resulting in what we commonly see as age-related health decline. While all bodies will sustain some levels of damage simply by being alive and exposed to countless varieties of stress, there are ways to mitigate the damage and keep your cells biologically more youthful than you might be chronologically. Sirtuins are very effective at keeping your muscles young, despite your age.

When you follow the Sirtfood Diet, you will be providing your body with everything it needs to protect against the damage that stress causes. Your cells will be better equipped to fight off free radicals and recover from chronic inflammation, which are both known to be root factors in stress and many other chronic diseases. If we can protect our muscle mass, we will also inherently be protecting our bodies against the ravages of age.

We can effectively sum up this section by assuring you that, the more you protect and develop healthy muscles, the healthier you will be overall and the easier it will be to find and stay at your ideal body weight. Sirtuins, activated by sirtfoods, are the easiest, most effective, and delicious way to accomplish this.

Sirtuins and Muscle Mass

Sirtuins help the body retain muscle mass even when dieting. How does this work? Well, sirtuins are a group of proteins with different effects. Sirt-1 is the protein responsible for causing the body to burn fat rather than muscle for energy, which is obviously a miracle for weight loss. Another useful aspect of Sirt-1 is its ability to improve skeletal muscle.

Skeletal muscle is all the muscles you voluntarily control, such as the muscles in your limbs, back, shoulders, and so on. There are two other types, cardiac muscle is what the heart is formed of, whilst smooth muscle is your involuntary muscles – which includes muscles around your blood vessels, face, and various parts of organs and other tissues.

Skeletal muscle is separated into two different groups, the blandly named type-1, and type-2. Type 1 muscle is effective at continued, sustained activity whereas type-2 muscle is effective at short, intense periods of activity. So, for example, you would predominantly use type-1 muscles for jogging, but type-2 muscles for sprinting.

Sirt-1 protects the type-1 muscles, but not the type-2 muscle, which is still broken down for energy. Therefore, holistic muscle mass drops when fasting, even though type-1 skeletal muscle mass increases.

Sirt-1 also influences how the muscles actually work. Sirt-1 is produced by the muscle cells, but the ability to produce Sirt-1 decreases as the muscle ages. As a result, muscle is harder to build as you age and doesn't grow as fast in response to exercise. A lack of sirt-1 also causes the muscles to become tired quicker and gradually decline over time.

When you start to consider these effects of Sirt-1, you can start to form a picture about why fasting helps keep the body supple. Fasting releases Sirt-1, which in turn helps skeletal muscle grow and stay in good shape. Sirt-1 is also released by consuming sirtuin activators, giving the Sirtfood Diet its muscle retaining power.

Sirtfoods and Your Diet

By now, we have talked about how sirtuins are proteins produced by genes in our body, which demonstrate numerous beneficial effects on the body. We all have noted three primary means of causing sirtuins to be released in the body: eating to a calorie deficit, stringent fasting, and exercise.

One of the primary claims of the Sirtfood Diet is that sirtuins can also be released through your diet, with the most potent sirtuin-releasing foods nicknamed Sirtfoods. Let us examine this claim in more detail.

It is known that a nutritionally rich diet, especially a diet high in fruit and vegetables, drastically reduces the risk of cancer and a legion of diseases. The reason why this is true has been attributed to many different factors, such as the increasingly popular 'anti-oxidants' as well as higher levels of minerals and vitamins in these foods.

Yet this isn't the rationale of why the Sirtfood Diet advocates so many plants and vegetables. Instead, the argument rests upon Sirtfoods being special, above and beyond all other components of our food. This argument actually rests upon the toxic qualities of the Sirtfoods, rather than their nutritional superiority.

Now, this is perhaps the most fascinating aspect of the Sirtfood Diet. The two authors of this diet argue that all the things we associate with improving our health (exercise, fasting, calorie restriction) all have a minor stress component. Essentially these activities put the body into a minor state of stress, causing the body to enact processes that help us adapt and improve.

This concept is called 'hormesis' and is basically the idea of what doesn't kill you, makes you stronger. Or in more scientific terms, small doses of certain harmful substances can produce a positive effect via the triggering of biological adaptations.

Plants themselves can have hormesis reactions to stressors in their environment. In fact, plant hormesis is rather sophisticated and plants, being stationary, have much more nuanced and varied stress reactions than mammals and humans. The reason why this is relevant is that when we ingest these plant foods, their stress reactions in the form of chemicals and hormones, we also ingest.

To bring it all together, eating these hormones and chemicals from 'stressed' plants can also benefit us, as some of our biological adaptations involve the usage of the same chemicals and hormones. In particular, polyphenols are known to benefit the human body and trigger sirtuin release.

This concept of using plants' stress-reactions to benefit our own is a field of study called xenohormesis. This is the very basis of Sirtfoods; sirtfoods are good for us because they contain sirtuins.

Chapter 4.   Live Longer and Healthier

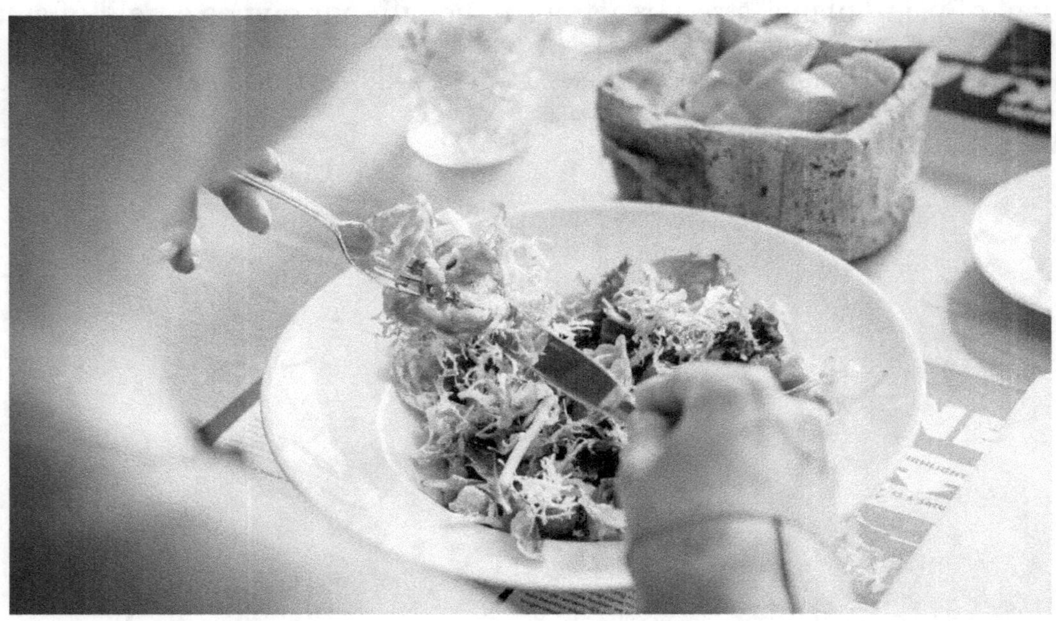

Tips to Build the Sirtfood Diet That Best Suits You

We have done something very unique with the Sirtfood Diet. We took the most powerful Sirtfoods on the planet and knitted them into a brand-new healthy diet, the likes of which were not seen before. We picked the "best and brightest" from the healthful diets we have ever identified and built a world-beating recipe from them.

The great thing is you don't immediately have to follow an Okinawan's typical diet or eat like an Italian mamma. This on the Sirtfood Diet is not only utterly unfeasible but also needless. Yes, one thing you may be taken by from the Sirtfoods list is their similarity. While you do not consume any of the items on the list at the moment, you are very much probably eating others. And why don't you just lose weight already?

The issue is addressed when we analyze the various elements that the most chopping-edge nutrition science displays are required to build a workable diet. It is about eating a proper amount of Sirtfoods, range, and shape. It's about adding ample protein portions to the Sirtfood bowls and then enjoying your foods at the right time of day.

And it's about the freedom to eat the genuinely savory foods you love in the quantities you admire.

Hitting Your Quota

Most people just don't eat nearly sufficient Sirtfoods right now to evoke a strong fat-burning and fitness-boosting influence. When the study looked at the utilization in the US diet of five main sirtuin-activating components (quercetin, luteolin, myricetin, kaempferol, and apigenin), human dietary intakes were found to be miserably thirteen milligrams a day. Conversely, the Japanese daily consumption was 5 times greater. Contrasting that with our Sirtfood Diet experiment, where everyday persons ate hundreds of milligrams of sirtuin-activating foods.

All we are speaking about is a true diet transformation in which we raise by as much as 50 times our daily consumption of sirtuin-activating components. Although that might seem overwhelming or unrealistic, it isn't necessarily. By taking all our highest level Sirtfoods and trying to put them together in a manner that is fully consistent with your stressful schedule, you can indeed efficiently and cheaply reach the level of consumption needed to gain all of the advantages.

The Power of Synergy

We think it is important to eat a vast array of these wonder nutrients as organic whole foods, where they coexist along with the dozens of other natural biologically active substances that work synergistically to increase our wellbeing. We think working with the natural world is best, instead of against. This is for this purpose that single nutrient supplementation does not display permanent effect time and time again, but the same component is represented in the form of an entire diet.

Take, for example, the basic component resveratrol which activates sirtuin. This is partially consumed in supplementary form, but its bioavailability (how much more the individual can use) is at least 6 times higher in its normal food material of red wine. Refer to this the reality that red wine produces not only one but a complete variety of sirtuin-activating polyphenols that work with each other to offer positive effects, like myricetin, piceatannol, quercetin, and epicatechin. Perhaps we could direct our focus from the turmeric to curcumin. Curcumin is very well-established as the main sirtuin-activating ingredient in turmeric, but work reveals that this whole turmeric has stronger PPAR-ÿ action to combat fat burning and is much more capable of suppressing cancer and decreasing blood glucose levels than isolated curcumin. It's not hard to understand that trying to isolate a single nutrient in its full food process is still nowhere near as successful as eating it.

Yet when we begin combining multiple Sirtfoods, what really makes a nutritional plan special is. For example, by trying to introduce it in quercetin-rich Sirtfoods we enhance the impacts of resveratrol-containing foods a lot further. Not even just that even in their conduct they complement one another. All of those are fat blockers, but how either of them actually achieves that is complicated. Resveratrol is very effective in promoting the deterioration of mature fat cells, while quercetin is active in preventing new fat tissue from developing. In addition, they ingest food on both ends, leading to a high losing weight impact than consuming just large amounts of a single ingredient.

So, this is a method which we see again and again. Foods that are high in sirtuin enhancer apigenin boost the quercetin uptake from diet and increase its function. Quercetin in effect has been shown to be synergistic with epigallocatechin gallate (EGCG) activity. And EGCG 's work with curcumin has been seen to be complementary. And so, it begins. Not only are individual whole products more effective than single ingredients, but we reach into yet another tapestry of beneficial effects that the natural world has blended — so deep, so pure, it's difficult to attempt to beat it.

Juice and Food: Get the Best of Both Worlds

Sirtfood Diet is a portion of both juices and whole food products. There we are speaking about juices made directly from a juicer — blenders and milkshake makers (including the NutriBullet) do not work. For others that may sound counterintuitive, based on the fact that the fiber is lost while it is juiced. Yet this is just what we need from leafy green vegetables.

Feed fiber includes what is termed non-extractable polyphenols (or NEPPs). Which are polyphenols, called sirtuin additives, which are bound to the fibrous portion of the food and only emitted by our helpful intestinal bacteria when decomposed. We don't even get the NEPPs by erasing the fiber and end up losing out on their righteousness. Crucially, though, the NEPP composition varies significantly based on the size of the plant. The NEPP material of a diet rich in fruits, cereals, and grains is meaningful and should be ingested whole (NEPPs provide over fifty percent of polyphenols in strawberries!). However, for leafy green vegetables, the essential compounds in the Sirtfood juice, they are much lesser even after having a bigger fiber content.

So, we get full value for our buck whenever it applies to leafy green vegetables by juicing them and eliminating the low-nutrient material, so we can use even increasing quantities and obtain an amazingly concentrated dose of sirtuin-activating polyphenols.

There is yet another benefit of cutting the fibers, too. Green leafy vegetables contain a form of fiber called non - soluble fiber which has a gastrointestinal scrubbing action. However, when we consume so much of it, it will frustrate and hurt our digestive lining quite as if we over-scrub stuff. That ensures that for so many people, green leafy vegetables-packed smoothies can overwhelm fibred, possibly aggravating or even inducing IBS (irritable bowel syndrome) and hampering our nutrient uptake.

When it tends to come to digesting their goodness, having a few of your Sirtfoods in juice form can even have significant benefits. For instance, matcha green tea has been one of the additives we include in the green juice. When we eat the EGCG sirtuin activator present in high amounts of green tea in the form of drinks lacking milk, its ingestion is higher than sixty-five percent. We also found it important to remember that transitioning towards smoothies to green juices carried about significant rises in their quantities of other vital nutrients, including magnesium and folic acid, as we ran lab tests on our own customers.

The core issue of it all is that to get those sirtuin genetic factors ringing for massive weight loss and wellbeing, we have to establish an eating plan that incorporates for greatest advantage both juices and whole meals.

The Power of Protein

These are plants that bring the Sirt into the nutrition of Sirtfood, yet to get optimum value,

Sirtfood foods will also have high protein content. It has been shown that a major component of the dietary specific protein leucine has extra advantages in enhancing SIRT1 to enhance fat loss and boost blood sugar regulation.

But leucine now has another role, and that's where it genuinely glows through its balanced interaction with Sirtfoods. Leucine effectively induces anabolism (building things) in our cells, especially in the muscle, which requires a great deal of energy and ensures that our energy producers (called mitochondria) have to work extra hours. It induces the need for such a Sirtfoods operation within our cells. As you may actually remember, one of the impacts of Sirtfoods is to increase the growth of more mitochondria, to increase their efficiency, and to make them blow fat as fuel. Our bodies, therefore, need these to fulfill this extra demand for energy. The truth of the matter is that we see a synergistic impact when mixing Sirtfoods with dietary protein that enhances sirtuin activation and eventually allows you to lose fat to support muscle development and better safety. For this reason, the meals in the guide are built to have a reasonable protein portion.

Oily fish is an incredibly strong protein alternative to supplement Sirtfoods' action since they are high in omega-3 fatty acids alongside their nutritional value. There is no way that you may have read a lot about the health effects of oily fish and especially omega-3 fish oils. And now new evidence shows that the advantages of omega-3 fats may come from improving the functioning of our sirtuin genomes.

In recent times, questions have been presented about the harmful impact of protein-rich diets on wellbeing, without any Sirtfoods to help counter the protein, we can come to recognize why. Leucine may be a knife with two-edges. We need Sirtfoods, as we have shown, to support our cells fulfill the metabolic requirements that leucine imposes upon them. Without them, though, our mitochondria may become unstable, so elevated rates of leucine will potentially encourage obesity so insulin tolerance, rather than boost safety. Sirtfoods support not only keeping the symptoms of leucine under control but also working effectively in our favor. Assume of leucine as tapping your foot on the losing weight and wellbeing accelerator, with Sirtfoods the device that guarantees that the cell fulfills the increased competition. The engine blew up, without any of the Sirtfoods.

Returning to worries about the safety consequences of protein-rich diets, the missing part of the equation is Sirtfoods. Usually, most nations diets are protein-rich but lack Sirtfoods to help counter it. That makes it imperative for Sirtfoods for becoming an essential component of how those nations feed.

Eat Early

Our ideology is superior when it comes to having a meal, preferably completing eating each day by 7 p.m. That is on two grounds. Firstly, to enjoy the Sirtfoods natural satiating power. Eating food that will leave you feeling full, happy, and energetic as you go about your day is even more effective than enduring the whole day feeling hungry enough to feed and stay full while having sleep throughout the night.

Chapter 5. Extreme Calorie Restriction and Extreme Exercise

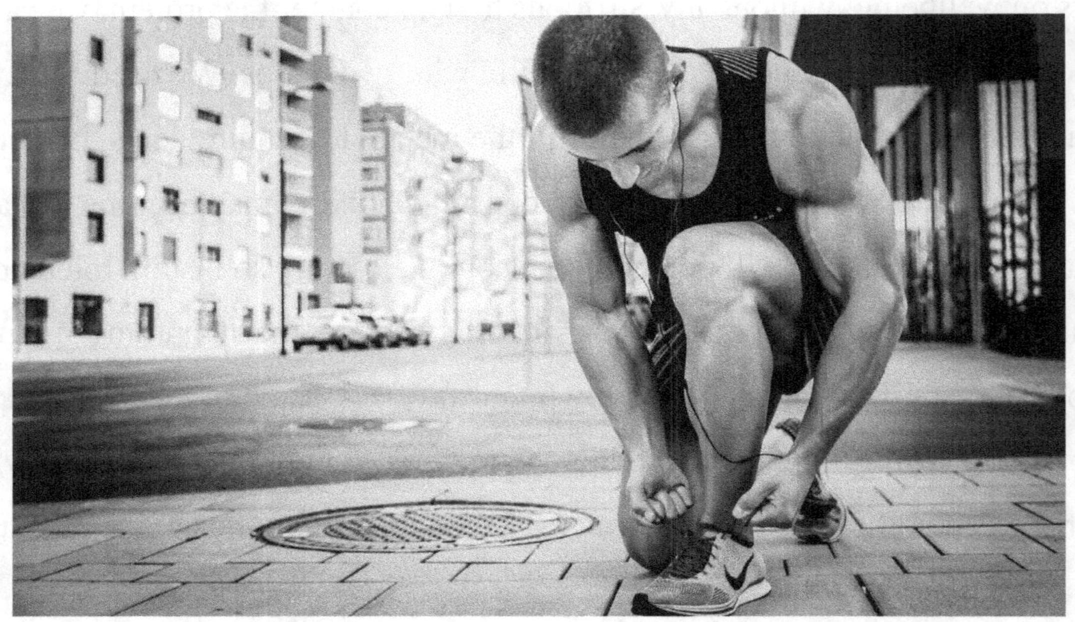

This diet makes the intake of food quite restrictive – focusing on counting calories and cutting out the major groups. Downsizing the portions to yield 1000 calories can surely make you lose weight drastically. Such levels of calorie restriction can anyways do that for anybody! This study, however, did not follow its participants after the three weeks to check whether they have gained back weight or not.

Your body uses up the energy from the emergency store like glycogen besides burning fat to provide you the energy that you will be required when you stop taking the necessary calories for normal living. Four molecules of water are required for storing one glycogen molecule. Using up this glycogen also makes your body release this water out of the body. Thus, by restricting calories in the first week, a fraction of weight loss looks like this: one-third from fat and the rest from glycogen and water. And your body will be able to replenish the glycogen store when you increase the intake of calories.

Therefore, you must follow this diet for losing weight as it can surely have healthy effects on your body. At the same time, you should also keep a check on your diet after the three weeks to avoid gaining weight unnecessarily as this diet is for an extremely short period and may not have a long-term impact on your body.

This diet can no doubt have a great weight loss effect on your body. Besides that, it can also aid other benefits of health because of the anti-inflammatory properties. The diet includes the intake of juice, which is rich in vitamins and minerals. But since it is only the juice, it does not contain the essential fiber from the whole vegetables and fruits. Above all, most of the foods that are included in this diet have naturally healthful properties.

However, restricting the calories to 1,500 per day will require the supervision of a physician as it is not for everyone. Sipping on the glasses of juice can also have effects on your teeth and the level of blood sugar. There is a complete chance that you have a deficiency in protein and other minerals. Side effects may include fatigue, irritability, and lightheadedness due to restriction in calorie intake. The first phase is nutritionally imbalanced and can have health consequences to some extent in some adults if followed for more than three weeks, however, it is generally not known to be dangerous for average healthy adults.

The Role of Exercise Along with Diet

Remaining healthy is at the highest point of everybody's need list, and our day-by-day decisions can decide exactly how healthy we are. Not all things are in our control, however, the propensities and approaches we take to our well-being can frequently have any kind of effect between being healthy and unhealthy. Two regions have the most power over our health, and those are our eating regimen and exercise. These both can easily affect our well-being and can play a role as being the primary factors in forestalling sickness and different problems further down the road.

Preventive social and health techniques like appropriate eating routine and exercise can likewise support your spending plan.

The most significant advantage of an incredible eating regimen and normal exercise is the manner in which it enables your body to fight off infections and different conditions. Your body's insusceptible framework is an unpredictable machine, and diet and exercise can vigorously influence it. An excessive number of intakes of inappropriate foods can put you in danger while the correct food sources, when supplemented with a workout, can really support your body's capacity to battle sickness. Both your eating regimen and exercise, particularly the latter, affect your state of mind. Synthetic chemicals in the cerebrum called "endorphins" may help you feel upbeat and positive, and these are activated by many types of exercise activity. Diet can have a considerable number of similar impacts, and there are many professionals out there proposing that appropriate eating regimen and exercise are two main considerations in generally maintaining psychological wellness. Both of them lessen pressure and can build cerebrum action. Endorphin incitement can likewise help forestall melancholy and raise confidence.

Sleep issues are a worry for many individuals around the world, and diet and exercise can impact your rest propensities. Exercise, specifically, can legitimately affect your capacity to nod off and stay unconscious. It's suggested that you don't practice vigorously or eat directly before sleep time, but appropriate propensities in the two zones can transform anxious evenings into delightful ones. If you are attempting to improve your activity and dietary propensities, it is best to ensure you sleep soundly every night.

You ought to focus on over two hours of medium-force exercise every week, or a somewhat low quantity of high-power work out. Blending vigorous exercise in with things like weight preparation or sports is an incredible method to change your exercises. Make a point to stretch out your body when working out and avoid potential risks.

Chapter 6.   Activate Your Genes

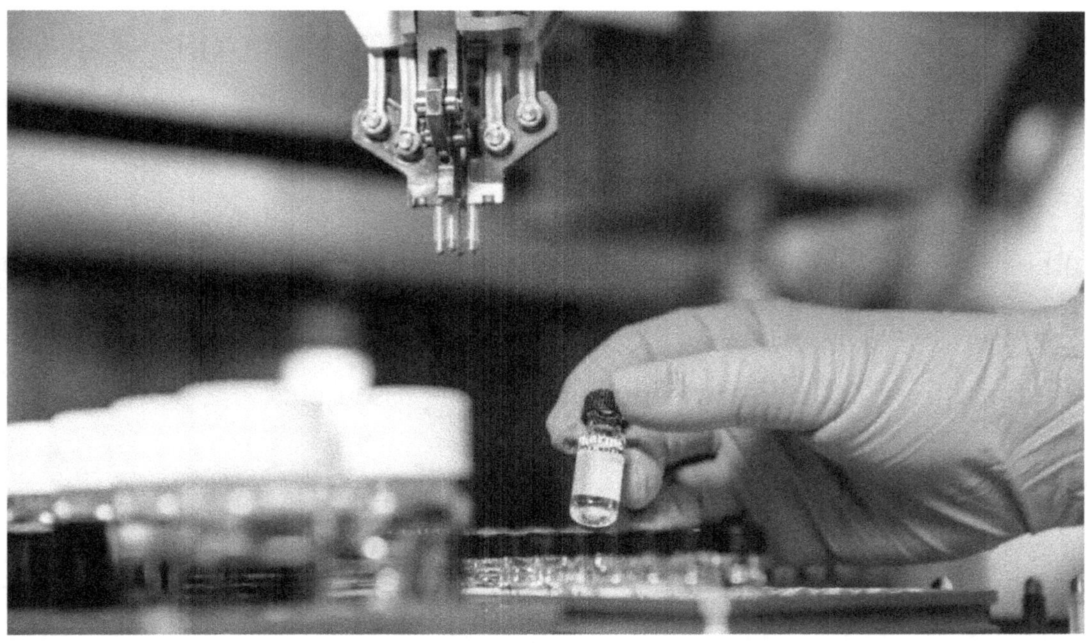

Sirtuins are also often called the Skinny Gene because of the role they can play in reducing human weight. But how these genes can make that magic happen is an important question. Biological sciences are not magic, it's all about understanding your body better and then meeting the body's needs to help boost its natural healthy activities. Similarly, when we boost the formation and stimulation of sirtuins in the cell, it automatically aids metabolism, prevents aging, and puts the body on a fast track.

Not every person is obese due to lack of exercise or the food they eat; some people have a naturally low metabolic rate, and it makes it almost impossible for them to get out of the trap of obesity. By stimulating the sirtuins, we can put the body on track and make burning calories faster and use them effectively.

Fasting-based diets have become very popular over the past few years. In fact, studies show that by fasting - that is, with moderate daily calorie restriction or by practicing a more radical, but less frequent intermittent fast - you can expect to lose about six pounds in six months and substantially reduce the risk of contracting certain diseases.

The accumulation of fat stops and the body blocks normal growth processes and enters "survival" mode. Fats are burned faster and the genes that repair and rejuvenate cells are activated. As a result, we lose weight and increase our resistance to disease.

The Mysteries of Thinness

Many studies have looked at the genetic specificities of overweight or obese people. Sadaf Farooqi, a professor at the University of Cambridge, has chosen to focus on those of thin people. The following are stated in this research:

Slimming is linked to genetics

The DNA study confirmed the results of studies: certain genes have a role in the risk of obesity and have allowed new discoveries to be made, in particular, that other genes seem to be involved in slimming. The researchers gathered the data collected to develop a genetic risk index. "As we imagined, we found that obese people have a higher genetic risk index than people with normal weight," said one of the study authors. Conversely, thin people have a lower genetic risk index. 74% of the slim people in the study had slim and healthy people in their genealogy.

Target these genes to avoid obesity

"It's easy to make hasty judgments and criticize people for their weight, but science shows that things are much more complex, says Sadaf Farooqi. He now wants to push his research to identify precisely which gene influences thinness, this could help put the weight of specific treatment strategies for overweight people.

All this, however, has a price. Lower energy intake leads to hunger, irritability, exhaustion, and loss of muscle mass. The problem is precisely this with fasting-based diets: when they are followed correctly, they work, but they make us feel so bad that we cannot respect them. The question, then, is the following: is it possible to obtain the same results without having to impose that drastic drop in calories and, therefore, without suffering the negative consequences?

Although Sirtfoods are not a mainstay of nutrition in England today, the situation was quite different in the past. They were a basic element, and if many have become rare and others have even disappeared, we will soon see that it is possible to reverse the course.

For the first time, researchers have just highlighted a genetic cause of pathological thinness, associated with a risk of high mortality. These studies, which point to the role of excess genes in underweight people who have difficulty eating, are published on Wednesday by the British scientific journal Nature. The study, which involved 100,000 people, was led by Philippe Froguel Imperial College in London and Institut Pasteur de Lille in France, and the Swiss team of Jacques Beckmann University of Lausanne.

The Franco-Anglo-Swiss team had discovered in 2010 that the presence of a single copy of a fragment of chromosome 16 could explain 1% of severe obesity. A fragment of chromosome 16 is known to be sometimes subject to fluctuations in the number of copies of its genes. The vast majority of people have two copies of each gene in this part of the chromosome, one transmitted by the mother, the other by the father. However, about one in 2,500 people have only one copy, an under-dosage, and one in 2,000 has three copies or overdose of genes.

It now demonstrates that people with an excess of genetic material and therefore having three copies of this part of chromosome 16 have significant, even extreme thinness. They are up to 20 times more likely to be underweight than the general population.

Foods That Activate Sirtuins

Turmeric and Kale are Sirtfoods. As indicated by analysts, these uncommon nourishments work by enacting explicit proteins in the body called sirtuins. Sirtuins are accepted to shield cells in the body from dying when they are under pressure and are thought to manage irritation, digestion, and the maturing procedure. Analysts likewise accept sirtuins impact the body's capacity to consume fat and lift digestion.

When on a Sirtfood Diet, you have to make sure that most of the following ingredients are in your meal plan:

- Arugula rocket
- Bird's eye chili
- Blueberries
- Buckwheat
- Capers
- Celery
- Coffee
- Dark chocolate 85% cocoa
- Extra-virgin olive oil
- Kale

Perhaps, other people might be thinking, "What kind of diet is this? Red wine and dark chocolate? It simply doesn't make any sense." As it turns out, it does. Scientifically speaking, the ingredients above are the richest in sirtuins, so it is highly recommended to consume them. However, moderate consumption is recommended, as you don't need to get drunk on red wine to get the sirtuins you need.

Moreover, you don't have to consume just these ingredients, as there aren't too many recipes of food made only from them. After all, this is what the sirtuin diet is about: combining calorie restriction with sirtfoods, not just to eat food rich in this class of proteins.

Resveratrol

This compound is a natural sirtuin activator that is found in red wine. It works to slow down aging and to make you as healthy as possible. This sirtuin enhancer also activates the sirtuin-1 protein that also supports healthy aging.

Pterostilbene

This sirtuin activator is a compound that is found in large concentrations in food items like blueberries. It has a structure similar to Resveratrol, and in some ways, they have similar effects on the body. This compound also activates sirtuin-1 proteins. It also works to cancel out issues related to inflammation in the body. With this compound, the cells of the heart are protected by oxygen deprivation cases by activating the sirtuin-1 protein.

Curcumin

This compound is another sirtuin activator that exists as a flavonoid. It can be heavily found in plant items like turmeric. Curcumin works to support the expression of sirtuin proteins in the body. They protect the cells of nerves from severe damage by activating the sirtuin-1 protein too. They also work in processes related to anti-oxidation. Apart from sirtuin-1, this protein regulates other sirtuin proteins like sirt-1, sirt-3, sirt-5, sirt-6, sirt-7, etc.

Chapter 7. List of Nutrient-Activating Foods

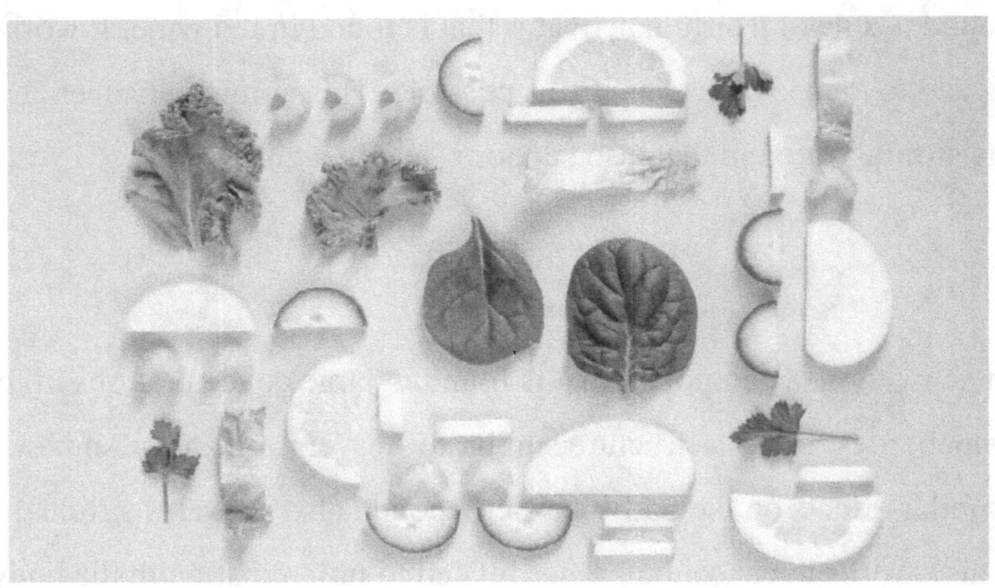

Green Tea (Especially Matcha)

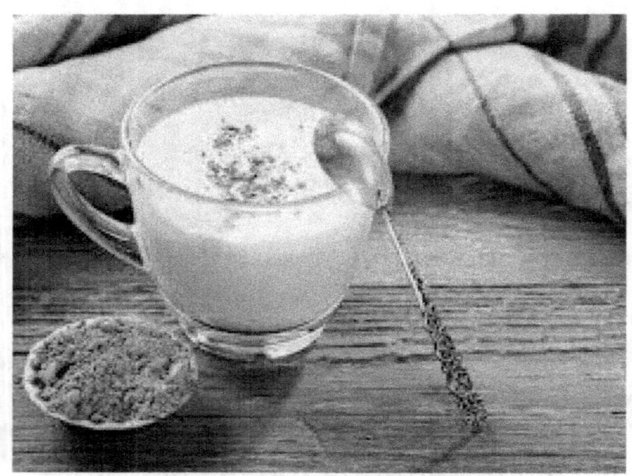

Green tea, or the Orient's toast, is becoming increasingly popular in the West and will be familiar to many. Like the growing awareness of its health benefits, green tea consumption is linked to less cancer, heart disease, diabetes, and osteoporosis. The reason it is thought that green tea is so good for us is mainly due to its rich content of a group of powerful plant compounds called catechins, the star of the show being a specific form of sirtuin-activating catechin known as epigallocatechin gallate (EGCG).

Garlic

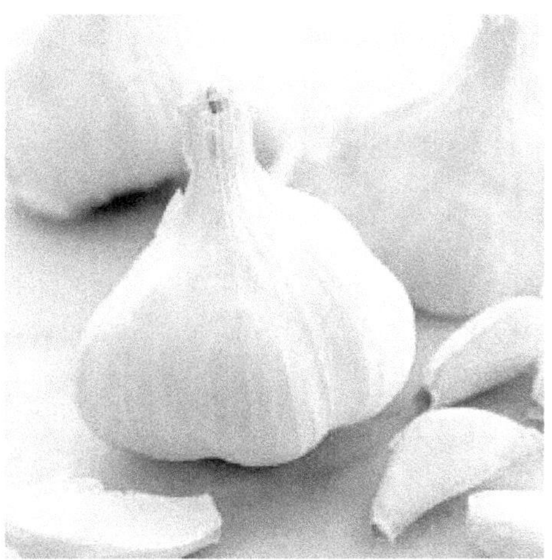

For thousands of years, garlic has been considered as one of the wonder foods of nature, with healing and rejuvenating properties. Egyptians fed pyramid crews with garlic to enhance their immunity, avoid various diseases, and strengthen their performance through their ability to prevent fatigue. Garlic is a potent natural antibiotic and antifungal that is sometimes used to help cure ulcers in the stomach. By promoting the elimination of waste products from the body, it can activate the lymphatic system to "detox" So besides being investigated for fat loss, it also packs a potent heart health punch, lowering cholesterol by around 10 percent so reducing blood pressure by 5 to 7 percent, as well as reducing blood and blood sugar stickiness. If you are worried about the odor of garlic being off-putting, then take note that when women were asked to determine a selection of men's body odors, it was found that those men who ate four or more garlic cloves a day had a much more appealing and friendly smell. Researchers claim this is because it is considered to be a stronger indicator of safety. Then there's always mints for fresher breath, of course!

Extra Virgin Olive Oil

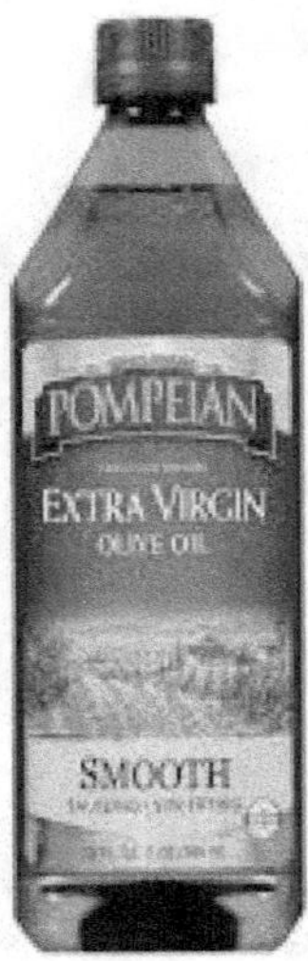

Olive oil is a traditional Mediterranean diet's most renowned food. The olive tree is among the world's oldest-known cultivated plants, also known as the "immortal tree." And since people started squeezing olives in stone mortars to gather them, the oil has been worshipped, almost 7,000 years ago.

Chilies

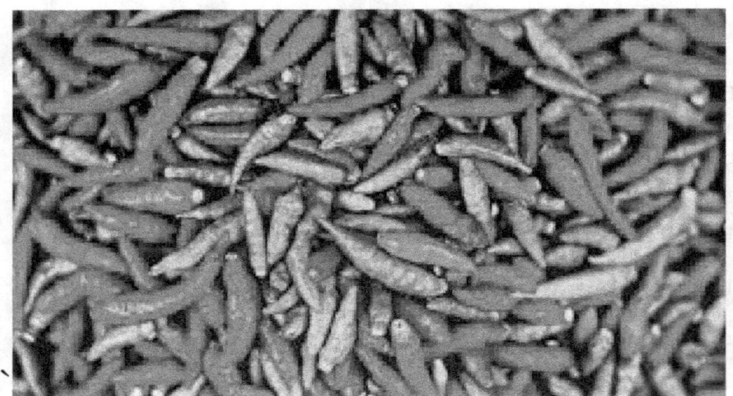

Chili has been an integral part of the gastronomic experience worldwide for thousands of years. At one point, we would be so enamored of it; it's baffling. Its pungent fire, caused by a substance called capsaicin in chilies, is designed as a mechanism of plant defense to cause pain and dissuade predators from feasting on it, and we appreciate that. The food and our infatuation with it are almost magical.

Red Endive

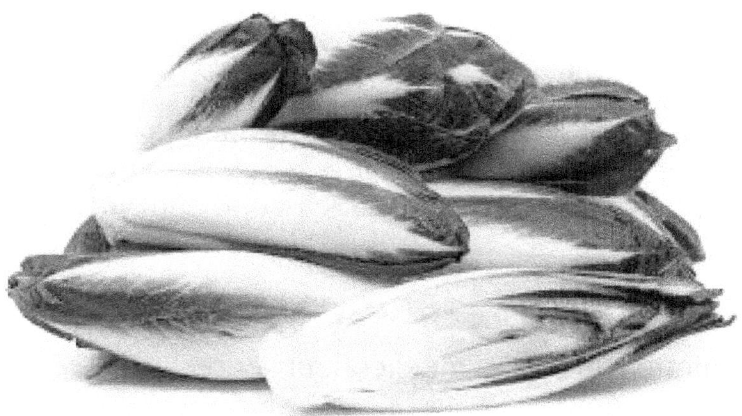

The endive is a relatively new kid on the block as far as vegetables go. Legend has it that a Belgian farmer found endives in 183, by mistake. The farmer stored chicory roots in his cellar, and then used them as a form of coffee substitute, only to forget them. Upon his return, he discovered that white leaves had sprouted, which he considered being soft, crunchy, and very tasty upon degustation. Endive is now grown all over the world, including the USA, and earns its Sirtfood badge thanks to its outstanding sirtuin activator luteolin material. Besides the well-established sirtuin-activating benefits, luteolin intake has become a promising approach to therapy to improve sociability in autistic children.

Parsley

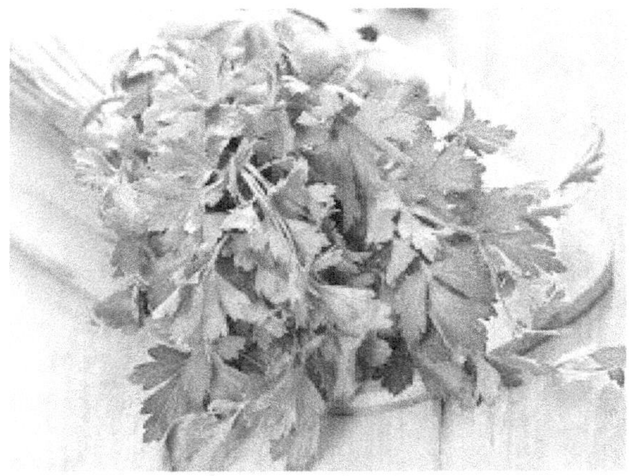

Parsley is a gastronomic conundrum. It so often appears in recipes, yet so often it's the green token man. At best, we serve a couple of chopped sprigs and tossed as an afterthought on a meal, at worst a solitary sprig for decorative purposes only. Either way, there on the plate, it is often still languishing long after we've finished eating. This culinary style derives from its common use in ancient Rome as a garnish for eating after meals in order to restore oxygen, rather than being part of the meal itself – and what a shame, because parsley is a fantastic food that packs a vivid and refreshing flavor filled with character.

Taste aside, what makes parsley very unique is that it is an excellent source of the sirtuin-activating nutrient apigenin, a real blessing since it is seldom contained in other foods in significant amounts. In our brains, apigenin binds fascinatingly to the benzodiazepine receptors, allowing us to relax and get us to sleep. Stack it all up, and it's time we valued parsley not as omnipresent food confetti, but as an in-house food to reap the wonderful health it can bring.

Medjool Dates

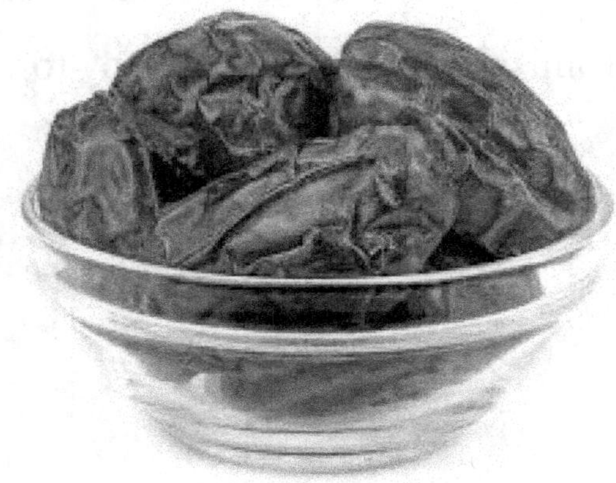

It may come as a surprise to include Medjool dates in a list of foods that stimulate weight loss and promote health – especially when we tell you that Medjool dates contain a whopping 66 percent sugar. Sugar doesn't have any sirtuin-activating properties at all – instead, it has well-established links to obesity, heart disease, and diabetes which is just the opposite of what we're looking to achieve. However, refined sugar is different from sugar carried in a naturally supplied vehicle filled with sirtuin-activating polyphenols – the date of the Medjool.

Medjool dates, consumed in moderation, do not really have any real significant blood-sugar-raising effects, in complete contrast with normal sugar. Instead, eating them is associated with having less diabetes and heart disease. They have been a staple food worldwide for decades, and there has been an increase of scientific interest in dates in recent years, which sees them emerging as a potential medicine for a number of diseases. This is where the Sirtfood Diet's beauty and strength lies: it refutes the dogma and helps you to indulge in sweet things in moderation without feeling guilty.

Kale

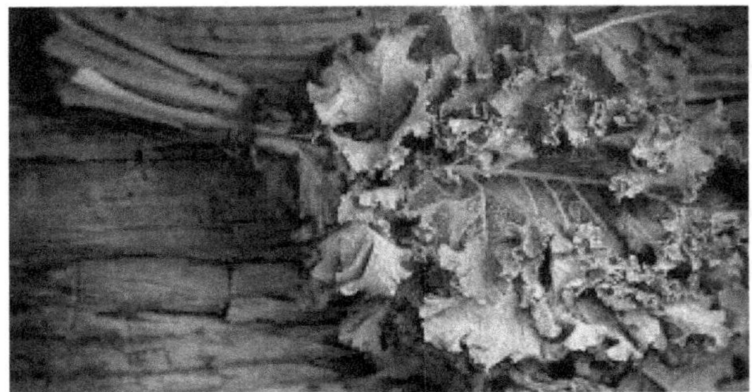

We are sincere cynics, but we are still suspicious of what drives the current advertising craze in superfoods. Is it science, or are its interests at stake? In recent years, few foods have exploded as dramatically as kale on the health scene. Described as the "lean, green brassica queen" (referring to its cruciferous vegetable family), it has become the chic vegetable for which all health-lovers and foodies are gunning. Every October, there is also a National Day of the Kale. But you don't have to wait until then to show your kale pride: there are already T-shirts, with trendy slogans like "Fed by Kale" and "Highway to Kale."

Coffee

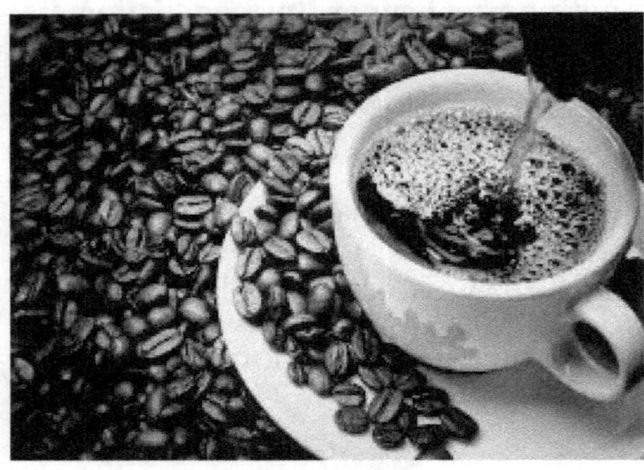

What's all that about Sirtfood coffee? We're listening to you. We can assure you that there is no typo. Gone are the days when a twinge of remorse disturbed our enjoyment of coffee. Work is unambiguous: coffee is a bona de alimentación. In reality, it is a true treasure trove of fantastic nutrients that trigger sirtuin. And with more than half of Americans drinking coffee every day (to the tune of $40 billion a year), coffee boasts the accolade of being America's number one source of polyphenols. The ultimate irony is that the one thing we were chastised by so many fitness "experts" for doing was, in fact, the best thing we were doing for our wellbeing each day.

Celery

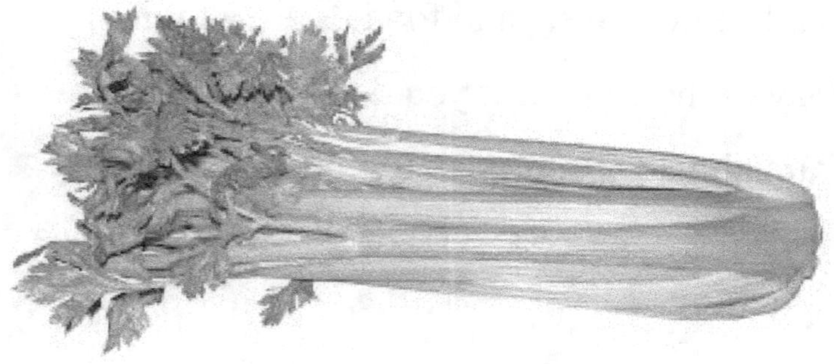

For centuries, Celery has been around and revered — with leaves found to adorn the remains of the Egyptian Pharaoh Tutankhamun who died around 1323 BCE. Early strains were very bitter, and celery was commonly considered a medicinal plant, particularly for washing and detoxification to prevent disease. The fact that liver, kidney, and gut safety are among the multitude of promising benefits that science is now demonstrating is especially important. In the seventeenth century, it was domesticated as a vegetable, and selective breeding reduced its strong bitter flavor to favor sweeter varieties, thereby establishing its position as a typical salad crop.

Capers

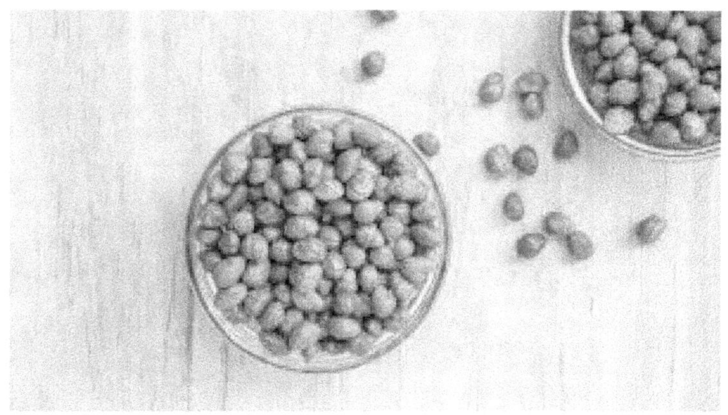

If you're not so familiar with capers, we're talking about those salty, dark green, pellet-like stuff you might only have had an opportunity to see on top of a pizza. But certainly, they are one of the most undervalued and neglected foods out there. Intriguingly, they are, in fact, the caper bush's own buds, which grow abundantly in the Mediterranean before being picked and preserved by hand. Studies now reveal that capers have significant antimicrobial, antidiabetic, anti-inflammatory, immunomodulatory, and antiviral properties, and they have a long history of being used as a medicine in the Mediterranean and North Africa. It's hardly shocking when we learn that they are filled with nutrients that trigger sirtuin.

Chapter 8.   How Much of These Nutrients Do You Need to Activate Certain Proteins?

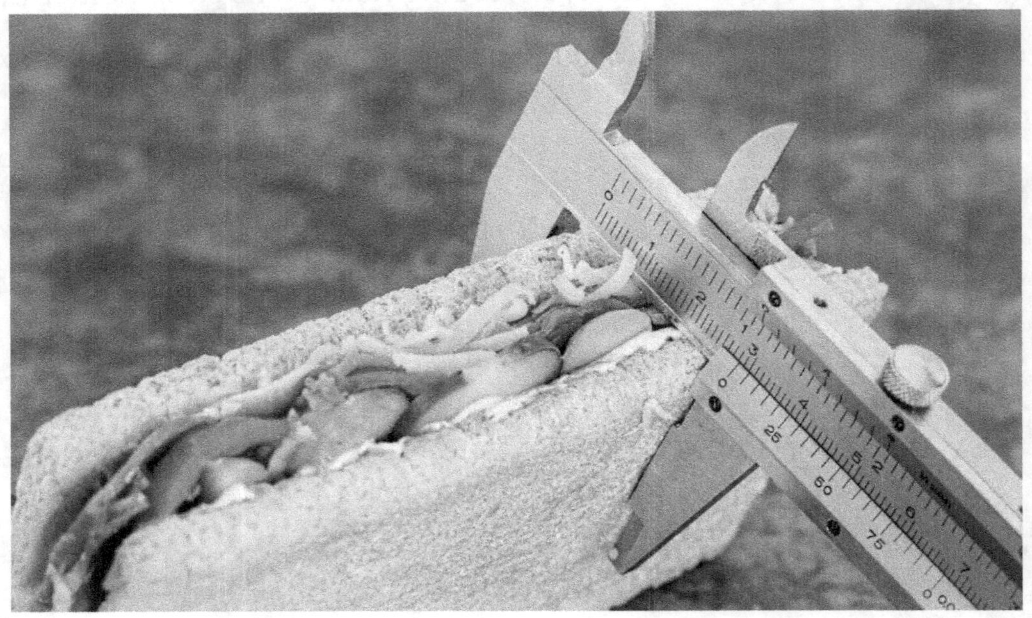

A day-by-day protein admission of about 1.0-1.2 g/kg of body weight is advantageous for stable metabolic capacity, as indicated by look into bolstered by individuals from the Protein Summit 2.0. That is, about 10% to 35% of your complete calories in a day ought to be protein, they composed.

Protein Summit 2.0 was a gathering in October 2013 of more than 60 nourishment specialists from the United States and around the globe to decide the ideal protein requirements for human wellbeing. It's essential to take note that the summit was supported by hamburger, egg, dairy, and pork industry gatherings. Yet, it brought about relevant reports that were freely distributed in an extraordinary enhancement to the American Journal of Clinical Nutrition.

A metabolically helpful protein consumption for an average grown-up ought to be 25-30 g for each supper, as per the Protein Summit's specialists. More established adults should eat somewhat more since they don't process protein just as more youthful grown-ups, they prescribed.

"Accordingly, unassumingly higher admissions of top-notch protein (1.0 g/kg to 1.5 g/kg every day), uniformly disseminated for the day, may maximally animate muscle protein blend, in this way adding to keeping up bulk in more established grown-ups," they concluded.

What Amount of Protein Do We Get?

Things being what they are, are Americans getting enough or more, to an extreme, protein? The average protein consumption for US grown-ups is 1.2 g/kg to 1.5 g/kg every day, or about 16% of their calories in protein, in light of 2003-2004 information from the NH (National Health) and NES (Nutrition Examination Survey). Even though these qualities surpass the RDA, they are well underneath the Protein Summit's upper scope of 35% of calories for protein.

Protein consumption changes with age, sex, and activity level. For instance, youngsters (ages 19-30) average 109 g of everyday protein while old ladies (age 71 and older) get around 59 g for each day, as per the information.

What Amount of Nourishment Is This?

It's hard for a great many people to picture in their minds how much protein is identical to, state, 0.8 g/kg of their body weight, or 25-30 g for each supper, or even 59 g for every day. Along these lines, here are a few models, as indicated by the US Department of Agriculture Food Composition Databases.

Can You Get Enough of Them from Food?

Yes, and it can be done only through careful and selective grocery shopping. Prepare a list of the ingredients that contain a high amount of sirtuins and check their utility as per your meal plan. There are certain ingredients like coffee, parsley, red wine, and chocolate, that you can have all the time. Make sure to stock up your kitchen cabinets with these ingredients.

Chapter 9.   Beyond the Diet: Your Personal Health Goals

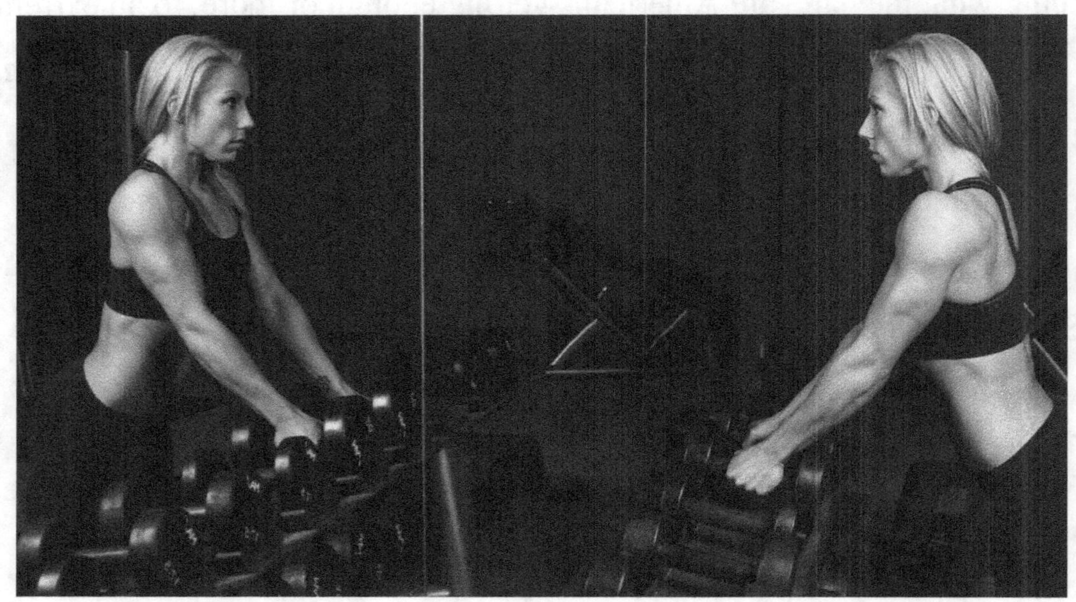

It is believed to be a healthy choice when we choose a diet that has the foods loaded with nutrients and also plays great roles in preventing aging or increasing lifespan (still not sure but evidence leads towards its positive effects) and reducing risky diseases like that of the heart and the body. It is mainly because of the existence of the antioxidants in these plant compounds, and most of them have anti-inflammatory properties.

Your body needs various types of foods to meet its nutrient requirements. Feeding only on a handful of them can never help your body to meet its requirements because it's a system that is to be fed with a variety of nutrients to keep it working.

Although the diet is filled with nutritious fruits and vegetables, it is unnecessarily restrictive in many of the other nutrients that are equally essential to keep the body functioning. To date, no unique and clear benefits of consuming this diet have been found over the other weight-loss diets. In addition to these restrictions, this diet allows you to consume only a thousand calories per day, which is not to be followed without the consultation of physicians. As the diet gradually heads towards the end, a person is allowed to increase the calorie intake to only fifteen hundred. Increasing it by only five hundred is even restrictive for several people. This diet allows you to drink three juices per day. Though juices are rich in sugars and poor in most of the dietary fibers that are essential for the body, unlike the whole vegetables and fruits, which are packed with essential fibers, juices are still a credible source of minerals and vitamins.

Do you know that taking foods rich in Sirtuin have significant benefits for our health? It would seem, at the current state of research, that there are no contraindications whatsoever. However, it remains essential to reiterate the importance of a varied, well-balanced diet and the absolute need for a medical-scientific opinion, before embarking on a change of diet, because we may have prior pathologies that could suffer an increase in change of diet. It must also be said that a diet, however incredibly efficient it may seem on paper, is not a magic slimming elixir, but that as in any case of life, to get results, it takes discipline, knowledge of the subject, and perseverance.

Exercise remains something indispensable, both to lose weight, to stay fit, and have a healthy life. We, therefore, advise you to stop the diet immediately if you experience discomfort or situations that can endanger your own or someone else's health.

From the research conducted so far, another element that has a vital role in this Sirt diet emerges, namely Resveratrol, a substance present in red wine and capable of acting as an activator for Sirtuins and their fat-burning mechanism. A diet rich in Sirtuin and Resveratrol also manages to induce the triggering of anti-aging and anti-oxidation of the cells and promotes cellular respiration in the body. It is, therefore, going to fight against dangerous free radicals, which are responsible for many human diseases.

The latter condition can be mimicked by the daily intake of moderate quantities of red wine and foods rich in Sirtuins, such as those we mentioned in our book. However, we are advising you to moderate wine consumption, as well as moderation in following this diet, because your health is the first thing we care about. As Confucius said: "Moderation is the way to a long and happy life."

The Diet Structure

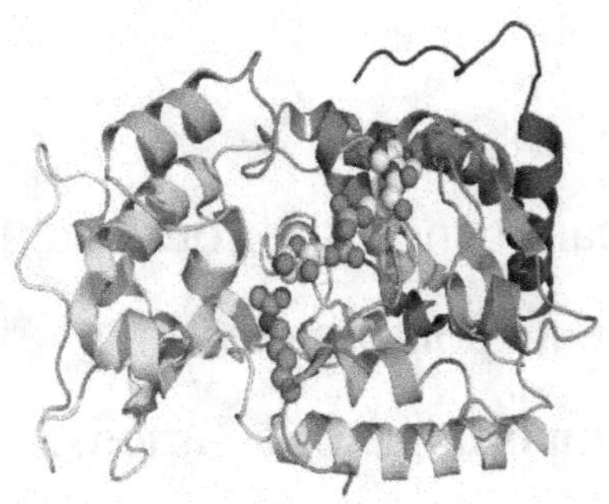

Sirtuins or Sir2 proteins constitute a class of proteins with enzymatic activity. The name derives from a silencing-regulating yeast gene, implicated in the regulation of cellular development. The research on sirtuins began in 1991 with Professor Leonard Guarente. Mammals possess seven sirtuins, which occupy several subcellular compartments.

Sirtuins use a very common co-factor, NAD, to achieve an unusual reaction. They take NAD, a co-factor used in oxidation-reduction reactions, and remove its characteristic nicotinamide ring. They then extract the acetyl group from an acetylated lysine of the target protein and transfer it to the remaining fragment of the NAD molecule. All sirtuins, like Sir2 shown above, have a common structural feature. They have two domains, one can bind the NAD and takes away the nicotinamide ring, the other places the acetylated lysine near the NAD and catalyzes the transfer of the acetyl group

The Role of Physiology

The activity of sirtuins is inhibited by nicotinamide. For this reason, it is hypothesized that the drugs that interfere with this specific receptor could increase the natural biological activities of sirtuins.

The mechanism of insulin that rises every time we ingest a sweet food or a refined food is the process that creates the greatest inflammation in our body. Raising insulin induces a resistance mechanism that over time creates inflammation in the tissues. An inflamed and therefore acidified tissue is the basis of every disease, especially cancer, and degenerative ones. Sirtuins regulate the metabolic processes linked to insulin resistance, have control over immunity, have a fundamental role in epigenetics, and are involved in defenses against tumor diseases.

Chapter 10.   Improve Your Energy Levels and Fight Disease

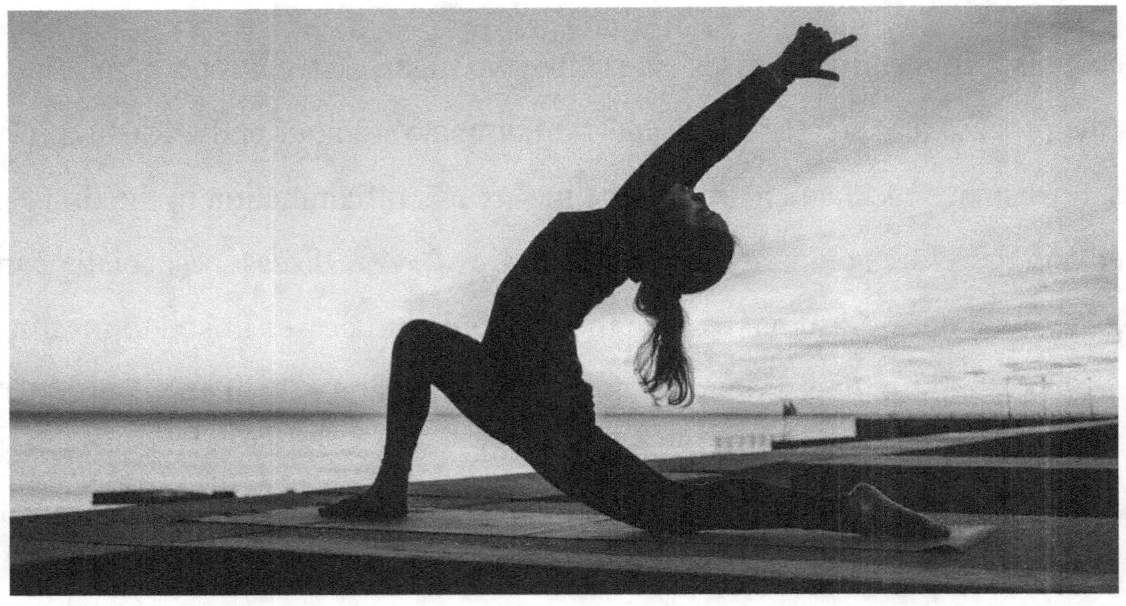

Sirtuins have a physiological duty in regulating gene expression and muscle differentiation by detecting changes in the ratio: [NADÿ]/[NADH]. SIRT1 suppresses differentiation of myoblasts by deacetylating and inhibiting the MyoD transcription factor. In skeletal muscles, SIRT1 organizes metabolic changes through the deacetylation of PGC-1a required for the activation of genes for the oxidation of mitochondrial fatty acids.

SIRT1 inhibits androgen and regulates androgen receptor function through deacetylation and transcription, thereby influencing muscle mass. It also acts as an important repressor of uncoupling protein-3 (UCP-3), which plays a role in protecting muscle cells against fatty acid overload, reducing the mitochondrial membrane potential, and reducing excessive reactive oxygen species production. In both fetal and adult skeletal muscles, SIRT2 regulates the cell cycle during cell differentiation. It also influences the dynamics of the microtubules by affecting the potential for redox.

Sirtuins and Fats

Sirtuins control a wide variety of processes, including transcription, digestion, and accumulation of fat, neurodegeneration, and aging. The various functions of these proteins were largely ascribed to their ability to catalyze the removal of acetyl groups from other proteins and lysine amino-acid residues through their deacetylase activity. Yet the sirtuin's exact biological action remains unclear. For example, one sirtuin, SIRT6 that has been involved in stabilizing the genome, inflammation, cancer-cell metabolism, and even lifespan is a very weak deacetylase. Surprisingly, the finding reveals that SIRT6 robustly extracts from lysine residues a myristoyl group— a long-chain fatty-acyl group. This biochemical action helps the enzyme to control the secretion of TNF-α, a cytokine protein produced from cells throughout inflammation. Stimulating sirtuins is also known as the vitamin niacin. Often closely related to sirtuin production are Plant substances such as quercetin (a bioflavonoid), resveratrol (a commonly found stilbenoid in grapes), and its chemical substance parents, pterostilbenes. If you don't have to starve after a Sirt food diet to trigger your endogenous sirtuins, you just need to eat the right food. The best part is, in moderation, you can always enjoy things like chocolate and red wine.

Nutritional supplements that contain niacin can also affect sirtuin activity and help you survive the surprises of life with much energy to spare. Sirtfoods are a newly discovered group of food, described as "particularly rich in special nutrients that can activate in our body the same skinny genes that fasting does when we consume them." These "skinny genes" are known as sirtuins, a class of proteins which research has demonstrated to be important in regulating biological pathways that affect our health and weight.

Fatty acids are taken up by transporters of fatty acids by the cell and then transported to mitochondria, where their oxidation contributes to ATP production. To generate ketone bodies, HMGCS2 breaks down the fatty acids. In the cytosol, lipogenesis (dashed arrows) assists in the synthesis of malonyl CoA fatty acids by fatty acid synthase, after which they are processed into triglycerides. When the energy demand is high, lipolysis will break down triglycerides to release fatty acids, mostly in fat tissue. Instead, these are absorbed into the bloodstream. SIRT6 represses gene expression involved in the synthesis of fatty acids.

Lipid Metabolism

SIRT1 regulates a series of lipid-metabolism related proteins and genes. A metabolic shift from lipid combination and storage to lipolysis is observed under the condition of fasting or short-term food deprivation, the features of which include decreased levels of ATP and NADH. With further research, under the fasting condition, the detailed mechanism related to how SIRT1 exerts its impact on lipid metabolism in these two processes is discussed separately in the following sense.

Lipids Synthesis.

SIRT1 is shown to play a role in the downregulation of both SREBP-1 and SREBP-2 during fasting, which results in lipid synthesis inhibition and fat storage. Until activation, SREBPs remain attached to the nuclear envelope and endoplasmic reticulum membranes. SREBPs undergo cleavage-induced activation and translocation to the nucleus when cellular sterol levels are low and promote the transcription of enzymes that are important for sterol biosynthesis. Additionally, resveratrol activation of SIRT1 correlates with the increase of AMP-activated protein kinase (AMPK), a nutrient-sensing molecule that inhibits the synthesis of fatty acid.

Lipolysis

In white adipose tissue, SIRT1's role is to keep back PPARπ activity by docking co-repressors, nuclear receptor co-repressor (NCoR), and retinoid and thyroid hormone receptor (SMRT) silencing mediator. The SIRT1/PPARπ/NCoR complex is recruited in the promoter region of target genes for specific DNA sequences and inhibits their transcription. This action can have negative effects on genes involved in the accumulation of fatty acids and the promotion of lipolysis. By favoring energy movement from white adipose tissue and oxidation in tissues such as brown adipose tissue, SIRT1 can alter the status of cellular energy production. Additionally, SIRT1 may be induced to activate fatty acid oxidation genes in the fasting liver, and PGC-1α deacetylates, which promote the use of fatty acids.

Cholesterol Transport

SIRT1 encourages survival in organisms ranging from yeast to mammals, and these defensive acts are thought to derive, at least in part, from beneficial energy control and metabolic homeostasis. High cholesterol levels have a significant impact on mortality, and a recent study indicates a correlation between cholesterol and SIRT1, which gives further indication of the lifetime prolongation role of SIRT1. SIRT1−/− in mice showed significant decreases in total plasma cholesterol levels, HDL cholesterol levels, and triglyceride levels, indicating that SIRT1 is a positive liver X receptor regulator (LXR). SIRT1 deacetylates LXR on lysine 432 and then promotes its ubiquitination, resulting in the efflux of cell cholesterol. LXR activation is beneficial in that it not only inhibits the absorption of intestinal cholesterol and promotes the transport of reverse cholesterol but also exerts potent anti-inflammatory effects that involve trans-repression. Until now, it remains doubtful to what extent the LXR deacetylation mediated by SIRT1 can affect these anti-inflammatory effects.

Growing evidence suggests that SHIRT is a key regulator for the metabolism of glucose and lipids. Through its deacetylase activity, it can regulate glucose and lipid metabolism by deacetylating certain proteins. SIRT 1 may be a new therapeutic target for the prevention of glucose-and lipid metabolism-related diseases.

Sirtuins and Diseases

Sirtuins regulate multiple vital functions and are involved in some pathologies, including metabolic diseases, neurodegenerative disorders, and cancer.

The rising occurrence of obesity-related diseases, such as dyslipidemia, diabetes, cardiovascular and cerebrovascular diseases, has become a bigger public health issue in industrialized countries. Many therapeutic and preventive strategies have seen the light of day to prevent or combat obesity, but few have to get through the test of time.

Another observation that caught attention in this sense is the so-called "French paradox." First reported in 1819 by Irish mathematician Samuel Black, the French paradox alludes to the fact that the French are viewed as having a relatively low incidence of cardiovascular and metabolic diseases, although their diet is high in saturated fat. One of the primary factors leading to this comparative benefit is believed to be the heavy intake of red wine, which is abundant in polyphenol resveratrol.

In the meantime, it has also been well known since the 1930s that caloric restriction (CR) can slow the aging process and delay the onset of various age-related diseases, such as cancer, cardiovascular diseases, and metabolic conditions. CR extends lifespan significantly in organisms ranging from yeast and nematodes to rodents and monkeys. CR's beneficial health outcomes are remarkably similar to those caused by resveratrol in many animal models, indicating that the molecular mechanisms through which resveratrol operates are identical to those triggered by CR. It has been proposed recently that the sirtuins could be the specific mediators that explain both the effects of CR pathways and resveratrol. In this appraisal, we will talk about the molecular mechanism underlying these sirtuins' biological activity, their functional roles in the physiology of the whole body, and their possible associations with human diseases.

Adp-Ribosyl Transferases or Nicotinamide Adenine Dinucleotide-Dependent Histone Deacetylases are sirtuins. The founding part of a group of the sirtuin protein family was Saccharomyces cerevisiae silent information regulator two proteins (Sir2p), a Nicotinamide adenine dinucleotide (NAD+)-dependent histone deacetylase (HDAC) that regulates the silencing of chromatin. Yeast strains with abnormal Sir2p levels exhibit defects in many cellular functions, including silencing transcription and recombination, senescence, and repairing DNA. To S. In addition to Sir2p, there are four sirtuins (NAD+-dependent histone deacetylases Hst1–Hst4), whereas, in mammals, there are seven homologs (i.e., SIRT1–SIRT7, indicated (Table 1). The remarkable preservation of sirtuin gene family members from yeast to humans indicates that these proteins are playing vital physiological roles

The authors of the Sirtfood Diet don't just claim that sirtuins can help improve skeletal muscle retention during dieting, but rather that they positively impact almost every dietary based disease in existence. For example, one claim is that sirtuins help improve overall heart health by protecting and strengthening the cardiac muscle (presumably in a similar method to how skeletal muscle is protected by sirt-1).

Another claim expounded is that the Sirtfood Diet also helps control diabetes. Some studies have found an association between Sirt-1 and the volume of insulin that can be released into the body. If you are familiar with the science behind diabetes, you may be aware that insulin is the hormone primarily responsible for controlling the levels of sugar in the blood. Therefore, by increasing the amount of insulin that can be released, sirt-1 can theoretically help tackle diabetes by causing higher amounts of blood sugar to be converted into fat.

On top of this, sirtuins have been argued to influence Alzheimer's. Individuals with Alzheimer's have been found to have notably lower levels of sirtuins than healthy peers, although the mechanism of action between sirtuin and the disease is not fully understood.

The authors of the Sirtfood Diet claim that sirtuins help prevent a build-up of the molecule's amyloid-B and tau protein, which is responsible for the plaques that form in the brains of Alzheimer's sufferers (and therefore all the corresponding symptoms). In fact, it isn't just argued that sirtuins help Alzheimer's, but also improves overall brain and cognitive function in regular people.

To add to the list of purported benefits is that sirtuins also help protect our bones. In particular, the specific argument is that sirtuin activation protects and helps retain our precious osteoblasts, which are a cell in our bones that allows more bone cells to be produced.

Finally, sirtuins have also been claimed to be a generic fighter against cancer, as they supposedly have tumor suppression properties. With all these claims, it is hard to discern fact from fiction. It does seem likely that a diet high in sirtuins does indeed have some of these benefits, but typically a diet high in sirtuins is more nutritious than an average Western diet. Therefore, it is not yet determined whether sirtuins are the active component producing these effects, or whether different molecules also present in sirtfoods are responsible.

Abbreviations

Aβ-Amyloid-β

AADPR-acetyl-ADP ribose

AASIS-amino acid-stimulated insulin secretion

AceCS2-acetyl coenzyme A synthetase 2

AD-Alzheimer's disease

GDH-glutamate dehydrogenase

HD-Huntington's disease

HDAC-histone deacetylase

MEF-mouse embryonic fibroblast

NAD nicotinamide adenine dinucleotide

NADH-reduced nicotinamide adenine dinucleotide

NFκB-nuclear factor κB

Nmnat1 Nicotinamide mononucleotide adenylyltransferase 1

PGC-1α-peroxisome proliferator-activated receptor γ coactivator 1α

PolyQ-polyglutamine

PPARγ-peroxisome proliferator-activated receptor γ

Sir2p-silent information regulator two protein

UCP-uncoupling protein

Chapter 11. The Changes That Last Are the Changes That Matter

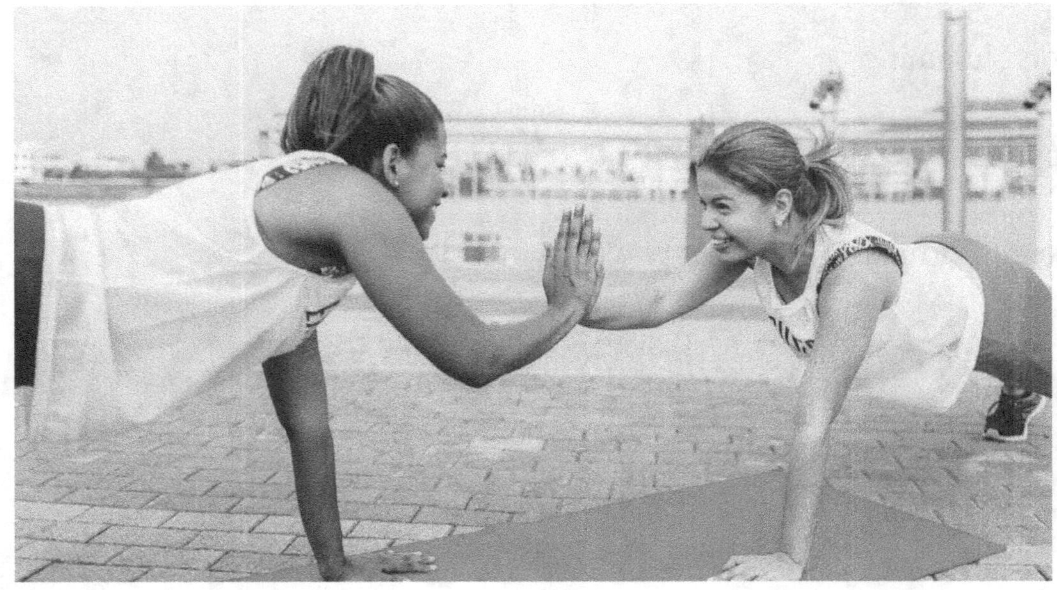

Do you want to have changes that last? Then below are a few things you should keep in mind.

A "diet" is nothing to be considered or frowned upon as a short-term fad. This should not be perceived as something that you are using for a "fast remedy" to a weight issue or safety condition. A diet would be a comprehensive lifestyle change, in a way, a thorough redesign of your eating habits. Your food is meant to become your way of life, a method of eating that you hold to for the long haul on a regular basis.

This should make it easy for you to be inspired and stick with it when you start talking about your diet this way:

Start Small

The first idea of having yourself on a diet is choosing to change your eating habits for the better. You'll need to give yourself a long-term dieting target. Say you want to become a full-fledged 100 percent vegetarian or vegan, for example, or you might want to eat only organic eventually. The very easiest way to get you started on your path towards reaching your target is to continue with tiny, practical improvements.

Take Baby Steps Daily

Now that you've settled on your long-term objective of dieting, the next move is to chart how you can do it. You want this plan to be mapped out one step at a time. Of starters, if your aim is to become a vegan, you can start by replacing a one-day meal with a "vegan meal." Alternatively, you can do something like having a single weekday, your "vegan day." Reasonably and wisely, choose your baby steps. It's certainly clear you can tell more about yourself better than anyone else, so you can make up your mind to start with either one meal or a whole day.

Stay Motivated

The best part of taking one-on-one baby steps is that this is what will help you stay motivated on your new diet plan. The trick to continuing on the path to dieting progress is to make practical improvements, one step at a time. Each time you take one of these baby steps, you'll feel proud of yourself, which will keep you inspired to keep going on and sticking to your diet schedule.

When you back up, meal by meal, or day by day, your baby steps slowly turn into leaps and boundaries. Before you know it, you should be well on your way to reaching your dieting target. It will be simpler and safer to stay motivated with every action you take toward your goal. The new lifestyle will become a "force of habit" when you get to the final phase of the plan.

Never Again Fail a Diet and Exercise Program

Why will too many diets and exercise plans fail to send in? What causes the rate to be so alarming? Was the system to blame?

Obesity is mounting at an alarming rate. Lots of people are experiencing major changes in lifestyle. Food routines are bought paying for Gym memberships, but after a few hours, and all diet and fitness plans have been discarded. Sure, the gym pass may not have been revoked yet, because they say that they will start exercising again soon, maybe!

What's going wrong exactly? Why are so many people quitting early? This lets people think it's just not worth dieting because they're destined to fail. One of the biggest causes, why diets fail, is that people want to see progress, 'Soon.' They're almost hoping to miss a few meals and 'Hey Presto' as if by chance all the weight is going to be gone miraculously.

Chapter 12.   Weight Loss and Your Health

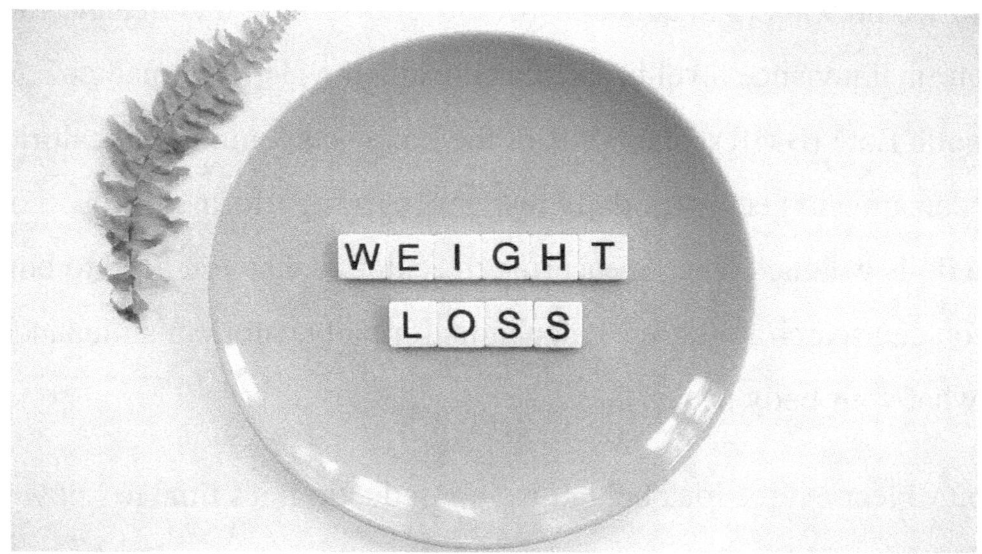

Experiencing difficulty in searching for a complete and accurate guide to weight reduction, search no more. This book will take you to a safer and sexier body with the best and most positive acts. Unlike other advice that focuses only on a single part of the diet, this book will feature all you need to know about weight reduction.

You must first understand how the body process works before entering into any diet or exercise program. The body has the ability to use a calorie maintenance level to perform its daily function. The proper number of calories allows you to walk around and maintain internal body functions. Calories are the source of energy for the body. You'll feel sick without the proper number of calories.

The calories that we need come from our eating and drinking habits. The weight does not go up or down because we eat the same number of calories that match our daily needs. Demonstrating this explanation: if your maintenance number is 3000 calories, and you eat the same amount a day, your weight will not be increased. Weight increases when we consume more than the level of calories we maintain. The opposite occurs when we use up the daily maintenance level, which is weight loss. We can also reduce calories from our daily maintenance level by eating less.

Therefore, an adult with a maintenance quantity of 3000 calories will consume 2500 calories to reduce weight.

I am sure you would want to understand your level of calorie maintenance at this moment. Your maintenance level is calculated using the Harris-Benedict Equation Basal Metabolic Rate (BMR). The BMR of the body is the number of calories that you need to consume to keep your daily responsibilities performed. How much exercise you do is weighed when measuring the calories that you need to burn per day. Also, you can search for online calculators for daily calorie maintenance level to understand what your body needs.

Now that you've learned the idea behind weight reduction, it's time to know the basic ways of weight loss. Those three essential ways are all you need. The first is to get to work out. Exercise can give you more calories to burn. Unless you stick to the maintenance level of your daily calories you will end up losing the same amount. So, no change in weight occurs. But if you'd like to reduce weight, you'll have to engage in exercise that loses a larger amount from your maintenance level of calories. You'll have to cut an additional 500 calories for weight loss with the last example.

You will also have to eat less of your daily maintenance number, apart from exercise. Those with a maintenance volume of 3000 will have to lose 500 calories and consume only 2500. There's a caloric deficit as you give your body a smaller amount of the calories it needs for maintenance. Engaging in more caloric shortages will cause a consistent weight loss for the body.

The best and most popular weight-loss method requires both diet and exercise. Eating fewer calories and burning more calories gives the body stability of what your activities are gaining and losing. It has been repeatedly established that you will get faster and longer-lasting weight loss results through a healthy diet and workouts. Using both approaches is also the best way and does not mess with your daily responsibilities.

Before jumping into a workout routine or diet, you must first evaluate the maintenance level of your body. The analysis will be the adjustment of your form toward a better routine. Start by regularly eating your calorie maintenance level for each day. Sustain such caloric intake for 2 to 3 weeks. It need not be the same number of calories as long as it is really close. Weigh yourself once a week (before eating and on an empty stomach) at the start of the day to ensure you are eating the right amount.

If you've had a steady weight for two to three weeks, then you've been able to eat the calories your maintenance standard requires. To lose your weight, you will eat 500 less of your daily maintenance amount per day. If your maintenance standard is 2500, you need to start consuming only 2000 calories per day.

Those who were unable to maintain their calories can still start a healthy weight reduction program. All you have to do is eat 500 less of your maintenance level and redo the body change with the reduced number of calories. If you have been good at eating the lowered level of maintenance, you will start consuming minus 500 of the initial number again.

To ensure you don't lose weight too fast is crucial to one. Reducing weight at a dangerous pace can threaten your well-being. When you find yourself consistently losing three or more pounds for some weeks in a row each week, then you will have to make some adjustments. The adjustment includes 250 to 300 calories to your daily intake. After that, with the new quantity, you have to start observing your weight. You shouldn't eat a smaller amount just remember. For enough necessary calories you need to exercise for a healthy weight reduction.

The speed of weight reduction prescribed is around one to two pounds per week. Remember, your body will not benefit from weight reductions very quickly. You have to maintain a loss velocity that will keep you fit. Much more important to your wellbeing than to look good. With very rapid weight loss our bodies can't catch up. In fact, if you quicken the procedure, it will simply change to stay alive. Instead, it keeps body fat so it can catch up. Then you just have to stick to losing one or two pounds a week. If you can do so for a year, you can eventually lose between fifty and 100 pounds!

Let's get off to the positive side. There's plenty of delicious food out there that still lets you hold and lose weight. Don't fall for fad diets that pretend low carbs or no fats will deliver the best result for you. Such diets are only out of your desperation to get income. All foods are required for a healthy physique. You just have to make them work accordingly. Doctors and nutritionists are the best experts to speak with on meal choices. They're giving your money value and they're just looking for your health.

A decent diet should include the right amounts of fats, carbohydrates, and proteins. An average healthy adult requires a fat content of 30 percent of their calorie intake. So, if you eat 2000 calories a day, you'll get 400 to 600 calories from fat. As 9 calories are contained in 1 gram of fat, the average person will need to eat 44 to 66 grams each day.

The best sources of fat are recipes for nuts, beans, olive and canola oil, avocados, fish oil, and flaxseed oil. Weight reducers should note that when it comes from healthy foods, fat really doesn't make you "fat." Fat won't get in your way of losing weight. It'll just add to your health and boost your stamina. As long as you get your fat from the sources mentioned, there's no need to worry.

Carbohydrates are another popular form of food for fad dieters. It is recommended that you eat 50 percent of your calorie intake from carbs. The ratio you have to remember: Four calories are one gram of carbohydrates. So, someone consuming 2000 calories a day will have to eat a thousand carbohydrates. Therefore, one has to eat 250 grams of carbohydrates a day. Fruit, vegetables, oatmeal, sweet potatoes, beans, and brown rice are healthy sources of carbs. To put it another way, eat complex carbohydrates rather than simple carbs. Simple carbohydrates come from a sugary diet such as white rice, white bread, soda, and other highly processed foods.

As for protein, for every kg of your body weight, the recommended minimum daily amount is 0.8 grams. Divide the weight by 2.2 then subtract by 0.8 to adjust for this. Since that is merely the minimum, people taking part in workouts should consume more than the calculated amount. To assure your safety you can eat a little more. Chicken, chicken, beef, lean meats, egg whites, nuts, and beans are the best protein options.

Let's go ahead with the meals that you must avoid. Obviously, most of those foods are very bad for your well-being. Soft drinks, fast-food, sweets, cookies, pastries, and chips are the things not to eat. Besides these, don't eat trans-and saturated fat foods. Stay away from the meals that have elevated levels of sodium and sugar. Generally, those meals are where you get your extra calories. You'll drive yourself toward an unhealthy lifestyle aside from the extra pounds.

Working out is the best way to have calories burned. It will also increase your strength, flexibility, and stamina in addition to weight loss. It will also help you escape heart disease and bone loss over the long run. For you to participate in 2 types of exercise: aerobic and anaerobic. Aerobic exercise has become more common as cardiovascular workouts. Cardio exercises improve your cardiovascular endurance, performed in moderate to average strength at a lasting rate. Cardio activities include sports such as walking, skating, jogging, swimming, riding, and using an elliptical machine. The most prescribed exercise in cardiology is one you enjoy, and you are eager to participate in as usual. Those who love walking should do a walk every day. While swimming is perfect for water lovers, bikers can continue with their pastime. The recommended schedule is thirty minutes, in terms of their time. Those still able to carry on above will extend it. The average person is however recommended for thirty minutes. Do aerobic exercise roughly three to six days a week.

Anaerobic exercise focuses on your muscle and endurance. They usually involve weight training, calisthenics (such as pushups), and the use of resistance machines. Anaerobic workouts are burning you a considerable number of calories. Although it isn't as many as cardio workouts, the cardio exercises will improve your stamina. It will produce very good appearances on your body, too. The muscle gain would make you look more toned and sexier. Anaerobic exercises advise speed is between two to four times a week.

There are also some diet legends that everybody should ignore. The first is the misconception of servings consuming fat and carbohydrates. Didn't we simply state that fat and carbs are necessary for the health of a person? You need those types of foods to maintain your calories. The next ones are those stupid and pointless one-meal diets. Eating just a little celery or cabbage soup just kills you. Only eating one tiny piece of food won't burn your fat. Your body will simply respond to food shortages and keep your current fat running.

Another myth is that workouts on spot reduction let you lose all your fats. The answer is not to focus on one single area. This is because you focus on your muscles during workouts. Unless fat wraps the muscles, they'll tend to be covered. You'll have to reduce that fat to show off your muscles.

Those products sold in infomercials are the most obvious fallacies. People don't lose their fat by relying on a single product. The same goes for those machines ab. These devices are just yet another example of spot reduction. Any other quick or easy means of reducing weight is simply out to get your money. You have to understand that weight loss requires perseverance and a substantial amount of time.

You should make use of a gym membership if you want to invest cash for your weight loss. The gyms have aerobic and anaerobic exercise machines. It is a powerful motivator, as well. You wouldn't want to spend your money and not take advantage of that membership. You're inspired by the people around you, too.

You need to eat smaller foods more habitually as regards your diet. Eating one to three large meals a day isn't recommended. Instead, break it up into 5 to 6 small meals. Consume the meals every two to three hours. Another way of improving your diet is to prepare your meals. Plan it for the start of the week and cook it early. This way, the unhealthy meals offered in restaurants or fast-food places don't bind you. You should also be taking water for your food. Drink this while you eat the meal. The water will make you full quicker and will save you from eating extra calories. Don't eat really quickly. It's going to take the body some time to realize that it is getting full. Gradually grind the food, and don't eat in a rush. When you eat too much, you'll be eating more than your body actually needs.

If you're just starting a routine on weight loss, you have to know it's a long-term activity. You will need to retain the weight by measuring your progress and making the necessary measurements. When you fail to do so, you're going to get that whole weight too fast again. Being safe is a change in lifestyle-a true commitment to the needs of your body.

How Sirtfood Can Help You Lose Weight

With the Sirtfood Diet, we have accomplished something exceptional. We've taken the most intense Sirtfoods on earth and have woven them into a fresh out of the box and better approach for eating, any semblance of which has never been seen. We have chosen the "most elite" from the most advantageous weight control diet at any point known and from them made a world-beating diet.

Without a doubt, one thing that may strike you from the list of Sirtfoods is their recognition. While you may not, right now, eat all the foods on the list, you in all probability are eating a few. So why are you not losing weight?

The appropriate response is discovered when we look at the changed components that the most forefront dietary science shows are required for building a diet that works.

It's tied in with eating Sirtfoods in the correct amount, variety, and types. It's tied in with supplementing Sirtfood dishes with liberal servings of protein and afterward eating your meals at the best time of day. Also, it's about the opportunity to eat the genuinely delectable foods that you appreciate in the quantities you like.

The vast majority of us essentially don't consume almost enough Sirtfoods to inspire an intense fat-burning and health-boosting impact. At the point when scientists took a look at the utilization of five key sirtuin-actuating supplements (quercetin, myricetin, kaempferol, luteolin, and apigenin) in the US diet, they saw singular everyday intake as scarcely 13 milligrams every day. Interestingly, the normal Japanese admission was multiple times higher. Contrast that and our Sirtfood Diet enlightenment process, where people will consume many milligrams of sirtuin-initiating supplements each day.

What we are discussing is an all-out eating routine transformation where we increment our day-by-day admission of sirtuin-actuating supplements by as much as fiftyfold. While this may sound overwhelming or illogical, it truly isn't. By taking all our top Sirtfoods and assembling them in a manner that is absolutely perfect with your bustling one's healthiness, you also can without much of a stretch and adequately arrive at the degree of admission expected to receive all the benefits.

We trust it is smarter to eat a wide scope of these wonder supplements as natural whole foods, where they exist together close by the several other regular bioactive plant natural compounds that demonstrations show to help our health. It's consequently that on numerous occasions enhancements of detached supplements neglect to show the enduring advantage, yet the same supplement, when given in whole food, does.

Take, for instance, the great sirtuin-enacting supplement resveratrol. In supplement form, it is ineffectively ingested; yet in its regular food network of red wine, its bioavailability (how much the body can utilize) is multiple times higher. Add to this the way that red wine contains sirtuin-initiating polyphenols, including piceatannol, quercetin, myricetin, and epicatechin. Or on the other hand, we may change our regard for curcumin from turmeric. Curcumin is established to be the key sirtuin-initiating supplement in turmeric, yet studies show that basic turmeric has better PPAR-γ action for battling fat loss and is progressively viable at contrasting malignancy and lessening glucose levels than curcumin. It's not hard to perceive any reason why disengaging a solitary supplement is not even close to as viable as eating it in its whole food form.

Be that as it may, what makes a dietary methodology extremely uncommon is the point at which we start to combine different Sirtfoods. For instance, by including quercetin-rich Sirtfoods, we upgrade the bioavailability of resveratrol-containing foods significantly further. Both their activities supplement one another. Both are fat busters, yet there are subtleties in how every one of them accomplishes this. Resveratrol is successful at assisting with pulverizing existing fat cells, while quercetin exceeds expectations in forestalling new fat cell development. Together they target fat from the two sides, bringing about a more noteworthy effect on fat loss than if we just ate a lot of a single food.

Also, this is an example we see again and again. Foods rich in the sirtuin activator, such as apigenin, improve the assimilation of quercetin from food and upgrade its movement. Thus, quercetin has appeared to synergize with the action of epigallocatechin gallate (EGCG). Also, EGCG has appeared to work synergistically with curcumin. In addition to the fact that individual whole foods are more intense than confined supplements, yet by combining Sirtfoods we tap into an entire embroidered artwork of medical advantages that nature has weaved—so complicated, so refined, it is difficult to attempt to best it.

Conclusion

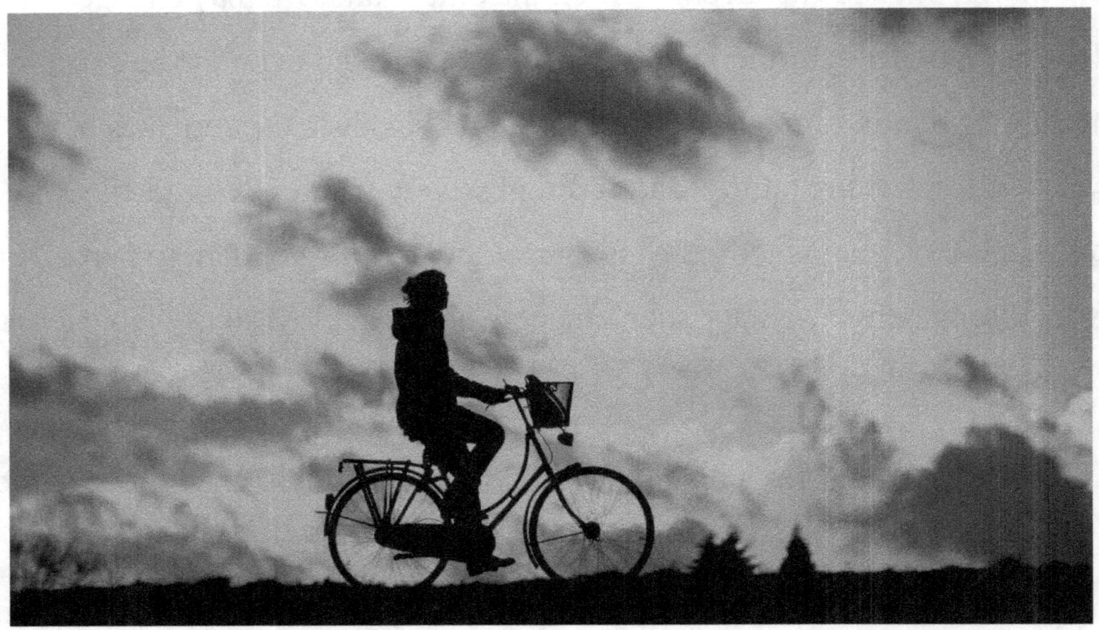

The Sirtfood Diet Cookbook has provided you with information about the diet plan and how to prepare meals that are easy to make and follows the diet's guidelines to living a healthier life with longevity and improved well-being. This will help you reach your ideal weight, just be sure to stick to the diet plan and avoid temptations. You can still treat yourself from time to time and eat unhealthy foods that you like but make sure to keep it at a minimum and continue to follow our guidelines for eating clean and healthy foods.

The Sirtfood Diet Plan is an easier-to-follow diet plan with its less extremist dieting guidelines and with its many good health benefits to give more motivation to stick to the plan. This diet plan has been proven effective through many repeated experiments. We have a lot of practical examples that provide you with information that indicates that sirtfoods can actually help you lose weight by increasing your metabolism and helping your body reduce the calories that are absorbed from the foods that you eat.

The majority of the food listed here are fruits, vegetables, and plant-based foods. Which are foods that you cannot go wrong with as long as you add other foods with sufficient macronutrients such as protein and carbohydrates. Just keep in mind to take your wine, dark chocolate, and caffeine consumption in moderation to avoid causing unintended harm to your body.

Finally, as a rule of thumb make sure to not put 100% of your trust in a diet plan with promises that sound a bit too good to be true. Set your expectations for more realistic results based on your current situation in life. Not everyone can live like Adele and other Sirtfood Diet celebrity endorsers.

The menu plan that is provided in this book will help you get on your feet. Whether you choose to use the plan exactly how I designed, customize it, or create your own from scratch, you will find that by having a plan and guide to follow eating healthier, losing weight, and boosting your health can be easier than ever. It's about time to give all the Sirtfood recipes from this book a try and see the results for yourself to prove that the Sirtfood Diet plan is a plan that is easy to follow and easy to stick with.

Now that you have learned all the things you need to know about The Sirtfood Diet Plan, go out there and use them to start living a healthier life to not only look better but also to feel better. You can also recommend this diet plan to your friends or family that you think will benefit from having a healthier lifestyle.